The Therapeutic Relationship in Complementary Health Care

To Annie's parents, Ruth and Fallas, and to her children, Hannah and Sam.

For Churchill Livingstone:

Senior Commissioning Editor: Inta Ozols
Project Manager: Valerie Burgess
Project Editor: Dinah Thom
Copy Editor: Holly Regan-Jones
Indexer: Liz Grainger
Design Direction: Judith Wright
Sales Promotion Executive: Hilary Brown

The Therapeutic Relationship in Complementary Health Care

Annie Mitchell BSc MA MSc CPsychol
Lecturer in Clinical and Community Psychology, Department of Psychology, Washington Singer Laboratories, University of Exeter, Exeter, UK

Maggie Cormack BA MA MPsychol PhD AFBPsS CPsychol
Honorary Research Fellow, Department of Psychology, Washington Singer Laboratories, University of Exeter, Exeter, UK

Foreword by

David Reilly FRCP MRCP FFHOM
Lead Consultant Physician, Glasgow Homoeopathic Hospital, Glasgow. Honorary Senior Lecturer in Medicine, The University Department of Medicine, Glasgow Royal Infirmary, Glasgow, UK

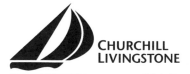

CHURCHILL
LIVINGSTONE

EDINBURGH LONDON NEW YORK OXFORD PHILADELPHIA ST LOUIS SYDNEY TORONTO 1998

Contents

Foreword

The title of this book belies its scope. In truth it tackles issues at the heart of all caring and service work, issues which bridge apparent divides between complementary and orthodox approaches.

The authors will challenge you, albeit in a scholarly and kindly way, to consider what you do give, and what you could give, over and above the specific intervention or service you provide. How are the human aspects of your work? What do you bring as yourself? Such challenges and reminders are perennially needed by us all, especially when human caring and professionalism are mixed.

Caring matters, and when we are unwell or not coping, or fear we are, we know this in our bones. This natural desire to help and be helped underpins all systems of care across time, culture and approach. As professionals we have a responsibility to give wise and effective support and guidance, backed up if need be by the symbols and substance of intervention. As patients and clients we must first ensure that these are on offer, and then bring ourselves with honesty to the encounter. When they are all present the capacity for change and support is great. But if the quality of these human encounters begins to erode then things crumble, in single encounters or whole systems of delivery, even if the offered interventions are appropriate and potent.

The dehumanisation of orthodox medicine stemmed in part from the delusion that technology had made caring redundant. What did it matter who gave you your prescription so long as it was 'effective'? The resultant separation of the carer from the person cared for in turn echoed the pre-existing idea of the separation of the patient's body from the person who experienced themselves within it. I believe this fragmentation is a key underlying reason for the remarkable rise in demand for alternative therapies around the Western World in the last 20 years. People have been seeking something better than a different, stressed doctor at each rushed visit. This is not self-indulgence, it is a prerequisite for a good outcome. While the debate around complementary medicine has raged about 'real' versus 'placebo' effects in these encounters, the central point has often been missed: patients and clients understand that effective care requires good human encounter every bit as much as good intervention. Western medicine is rediscovering that the one enhances or disrupts the other, the information often obscurely buried under the guise of terms like placebo, psychology and psychoneuro-immunology. Perhaps the greatest single contribution from complementary medicine so far has been the re-awakening of the importance of good healing encounters within orthodox care, yet, paradoxically, there are now signs that practitioners of complementary medicine are not championing this aspect of their work. In fact they are in danger of undervaluing it, drawn by the human tendencies to invest in the potency of their chosen intervention at the expense of their consultation—be that intervention an acupuncture needle or a psychological approach. The climate of demands from increasing professionalisation will likely intensify this tendency in the years ahead; the demands of survival and success, and of scientific and culture evaluation.

This work makes a timely and important contribution to the celebration and development of therapeutic relationships. Through history, literature review, and reflection it takes you to a working model of healing encounters, tempering the academic enquiry with the practical and humane.

D. R.

Preface

One of the many alarming things about writing a book is the air of finality with which the last full-stop is placed. For me, this is in contrast to the ebb and flow of writing, during which I experienced a variety of imaginary relationships with many possible readers, all mirroring the real relationships with teachers, students, colleagues, patients, clients and friends with whom the ideas expressed in the book developed. There is a continual tension, in writing a book of this sort, (and, indeed, in rigorous clinical practice) between the measured scepticism of the cautious academic and the enthusiastic conviction of the committed clinician. This tension is held in our need for humility in the face of our inability to plumb the depths of the many layers of reality, fantasy and imagination contained within human relationships in general and healing relationships in particular.

In many ways, the process of writing this book echoed the process of treatment which it describes. The teachers who first set me on the path towards becoming a clinician, Elizabeth and John Newson, instilled, at the start of my career as a developmental psychologist, a sense of the importance of mutuality, through their fundamental respect for the humanity of children and parents, however gravely troubled their lives and circumstances. Later, Jim Orford and Jim Drewery, teachers of clinical psychology, were mentors who tempered the potential arrogance of an aspiring practitioner with down-to-earth awareness of the limitations of professional expertise in face of the realities of human suffering. My introduction to the world of complementary medicine was through Roger Hill and Simon Mills who succeeded in creating a centre at Exeter where students from many traditions and disciplines worked to develop mutual respect for their very different perspectives. This context of mutuality provided a safe educational setting and an atmosphere of trust within which our careful attention to one another's ideas, knowledge and clinical experience enabled us to articulate our core beliefs about the centrality of the therapeutic relationship in healing encounters. All the students I have taught (orthodox and complementary practitioners) at the Centre for Complementary Health Studies have contributed to the ideas set out in this book: in particular Francesca Diebschlag, Kylza Estrella de Souza, Mark Kane and the year group of 1993: Vicky Foulger, Laureen Hemming, Sally Hill, Simeon Niel-Asher, Mary Bredin, Paul Coe, Margaret Gulliver, Catherine Littlewood, Sharon Lucas, Alistair McConnon, Jonathan Shaw, Serena Scrine, Simon Lansdown and Wendy Chamberlain.

I was also, while writing the book, engaged in working with a group of people who worked for, and used, the services of a local community health care trust: in a different way they too have contributed to this book through sharing their personal perspectives on what is essential in health care. They articulated and demonstrated the importance of kindness, tolerance, love and concern for one another. I am very grateful for the inspiration of (amongst others) Therese Canning, Gerald Conyngham, Pam Coughlan, Nick Lyttelton, Tom McCausland, Dave Rendell and Paula Teade. I have also been helped and influenced by the work of Joy Thompson, Aileen Knapp, Wendy Stayte, Simon Dudbridge and Malcolm Learmonth.

There were certainly times when writing a book seemed to be too challenging, and I am very appreciative that Maggie Cormack kept a clear vision of the importance of the therapeutic relationship, seeing it at the heart of health care and believing the ideas to be worth her commitment to working with me on the book.

Other friends have contributed too, (especially Shira Rub and Richard Lemon), through support and encouragement; in particular, many conversations with Mandy Cole, and some of her clinical wisdom (especially at the end of Chapter 7) have been incorporated into the book. Finally, I am grateful to the artist, David Davies, whose Vibration Picture (which I bought to celebrate completing the manuscript) is depicted on the book cover. I think that the picture's vibrancy resonates with the central notions of empathy, harmony and energy in complementary health care, and is a reminder that words alone cannot convey the significance of the healer's art.

We are only too aware of the limitations of this book, and this is the point at which the need for mutuality returns. Readers may be exasperated by our emphasis on the similarities between disciplines, perhaps feeling that we have neglected the many ways in which complementary medical traditions are as different to one another as are complementary and orthodox approaches within Western culture. We now need to consider further the special characteristics of the therapeutic relationship within each discipline, with specific developments of the model of the process of treatment, along with particular clinical implications developed by practitioners who have intimate knowledge of their own traditions. This book focuses on one-to-one relationships between patient and practitioner in very general terms: there is more to be written about the particular needs of different people and patients across the human life span: children and older adults, men and women, people from a range of cultural origins and those with specific disabilities and illnesses. Finally, we need to know more about our collective views and experiences of illnesses and treatments, and to develop outcome measures which reflect patients' (as well as society's, professionals' and academics') criteria for effective treatment, so that health care, whether orthodox or complementary, can be evaluated meaningfully as well as rigorously. Clinicians and researchers may be patients too, and we *all* have a stake in helping to develop health care which treats us as significant individuals and as interdependent citizens in our social world.

A.M.

A long time ago, the Centre for Complementary Health Studies at the University of Exeter asked for some help in putting together a module on the therapeutic relationship for its BPhil degree in complementary therapy. I took on the task and wrote an outline syllabus, which was adopted. Later, I started to do some teaching on the module, but realised that I had over-committed myself and that I could no longer maintain a high level of involvement in the course, given all the other things I was attempting to do. There was a sense of having fulfilled my obligation and satisfied my own interests by producing the syllabus and that it was now time for someone else to take it over. Annie was the person who picked up where I left off and not only taught the module but developed it well beyond its original shape, bringing into it a wealth of information from the experiences of complementary practitioners and framing it in a coherent theoretical perspective.

More recently, Annie embarked on writing this book, using much of the content of the module and incorporating the developed ideas of the previous few years. After some while, the task came under threat from other concerns and demands and nearly foundered. We discussed the difficulties and agreed that the way forward was to combine our talents: Annie's imagination and creative ideas with my analytic approach and attention to minutiae. Thus we combined the classic right-brain and left-brain skills in a way that felt comfortable for both of us, giving us mutual support and balancing chore with pleasure. As clinical psychologists, we were working together on the essential tension in our profession between the scientist-practitioner and the humanistic, interpersonally-oriented therapist.

Professionally, we are outsiders to complementary practice, but insiders in terms of some of the debates and issues. Clinical psychology is a small profession which has been accepted in the health care arena, working alongside traditional medical approaches. Our work involves much more than technique, focusing in large part on helping people to regain command of their own lives when it has been lost for a while. Thus, our concerns about the therapeutic relationship are those of discovering what patients want, understanding the personal meanings of their dilemmas, exploring how change occurs, empowering people in their endeavours and remaining sufficiently healthy and effective in ourselves to be of service to the people we see. These themes are addressed in this book in the context of complementary health care where we have set out some of the evidence and theory which has influenced our own ideas about how to make the most of the therapeutic relationship.

M. C.

1

Introduction: promoting self-healing through the therapeutic relationship

THE SCOPE OF THE BOOK

The purpose of this book is to help practitioners reflect on what they almost certainly want to achieve in their work: how best to use themselves to promote the healing of their patients. The book arose from a series of interdisciplinary seminars, initially devised by Maggie Cormack and then developed and taught by Annie Mitchell over a period of 5 years at the Centre for Complementary Health Studies at the University of Exeter. The students came from a variety of backgrounds, both orthodox (medicine, nursing, physiotherapy) and non-orthodox (including herbalism, osteopathy, homeopathy, Chinese medicine and many others). The teaching was informed by our background as clinical psychologists. We were particularly concerned to try to understand the core factors which underlie the help offered across therapies despite their apparent diversity in concepts and technique.

Participants in the seminars worked hard to reflect and learn from personal experiences as practitioners and as patients. Together, as a group, we found that our inspiration lay in trying to accept, respect, honour and understand one another's differing perspectives, styles and skills. The parallel for work with patients became clear: to be effective in our treatments we must establish a strong framework of mutual trust and care, within which we do all we can to grasp the patient's distress or disorder from his own perspective and then use our skills, knowledge and techniques in the service of his needs. The main message of this book is that the experience of a therapeutic relationship can facilitate change: relationships can heal.

As the book's title conveys, the main emphasis will be on considering the implications of what is known about the therapeutic relationship for complementary practice. However, much of the evidence will, of necessity, be drawn from studies of orthodox health care, including psychotherapy, as little research has been done so far on the therapeutic relationship in complementary health care. The research will be found to support the aspirations of complementary practitioners to make full beneficial use of the therapeutic relationship. The book is aimed primarily at practitioners whose disciplines come from outside that which is currently regarded in the West as orthodox, scientific or mainstream medicine, but we hope that it will be relevant to those orthodox health practitioners, whether nurses, doctors or other therapists, who wish to reflect more deeply on the nature of the therapeutic relationship than is normally encouraged in their basic education and training.

We must acknowledge the limitations of the book, which is largely focused on the individual relationship between patient and practitioner in complementary health care within Western culture. It is not about counselling, which has its own techniques and theories, although many ideas drawn both from the counselling and psychotherapy literature will be relevant to our search for fundamental core themes in treatment. Patients who come for complementary health care are not necessarily asking for, or wanting, counselling; indeed, many patients may have actively chosen not to engage directly with psychological or interpersonal issues and we believe that this choice must be respected. Nevertheless, we argue that psychological and interpersonal processes inevitably form part of all treatment encounters and that these processes can be used to the patient's advantage. Readers who want to learn more about counselling are encouraged to read further: Sage Publications' *'Counselling in practice'* series, edited by Windy Dryden, may be useful to complementary practitioners. *Counselling for psychosomatic problems* (Sanders 1996) is particularly relevant since it puts forward a range of techniques to enable the practitioner to help patients with chronic difficulties to make productive links among their beliefs, feelings and behaviours in relation to their illness.

At many times throughout the text, we will allude to our knowledge that illness, health and healing are all embedded in a social context which reflects cultural meanings and structural inequalities. People have differential access to the basic physical and social requirements for healthy living – wholesome food, safety, warmth, support, security and love. The medical epidemiologist Wilkinson (1996) has pulled together fundamental research which confirms that, in the developed world, it is the most egalitarian societies which have the best health and that societies which are both egalitarian and healthy are also markedly more socially cohesive than others. Social stress, poor social networks, low self-esteem, depression, anxiety, insecurity and the loss of a sense of control all contribute to a pattern of poor quality of life along with higher rates of morbidity and mortality. Ill health is greatest among disadvantaged people in those societies with the largest economic differentials between social groups. Wilkinson concludes that in terms of economics and health care, priority must now be given to the satisfaction of social needs.

It is beyond the scope of this book to elaborate on the political and sociological implications of the imperative to develop socially cohesive communities. The focus of the book is largely the individual relationship of one patient with one practitioner. Anthropology and sociology are only briefly mentioned in terms of framing the nature of the relationship. However, we do wish to argue most strongly that, at the individual level, the promotion of health and the challenging of disease, illness and sickness require the establishment of therapeutic relationships which provide social support and which promote a sense of personal power and control.

A note is needed here about nomenclature. We intend, throughout the book, to refer to the practitioner as 'she' and the patient as 'he'. This is in spite of the fact that we know that in both orthodox and complementary settings, women outnumber men as patients somewhere in the ratio of two to one. We hope that by referring to patients and practitioners as 'he' and 'she' respectively, this will promote our recognition that men (as well as women) *can* come for help and that women (as well as men) *do* offer help.

Women, as well as having to look after themselves, very often have responsibility for the well-being of the whole family: their children, husbands, partners. It has been argued that, because of the roles that women are traditionally expected to play and because of their relative lack of power in the world, many women (in common with others who are relatively disadvantaged in society) become acutely sensitive to social cues and interpersonal nuances within the relationships between themselves and other people around them (Baker Miller 1986, Rowbotham 1990). The issues and arguments here are complex and subtle. It seems, though, that the requirements for maturity in our society are often considered to include a capacity to be independent and autonomous and yet also to be connected with others. The opportunities to be independent and to be connected are differentially available to men and women and, moreover, are differentially valued within Western culture. Independence and autonomy tend to be valued more highly, at least in our society, than dependence and connectedness.

In the world of healing and medicine, the stereotypical female attributes of sensitivity, feeling with and for others, empathy and intuition have been both appreciated and recognized yet also viewed with suspicion and alarm, as evidenced, for example, by the occasional scapegoating of powerful female practitioners (Achterberg 1990, Brooke 1993). Prejudices and fears limit options and diminish potential effectiveness. We need to remain alert to the particular issues that face men and women as patients and as practitioners. These questions have been helpfully enlarged elsewhere (see, for example, Miller & Bell 1996, Ussher & Nicolson 1992). We would argue that the split in value and function between what are seen as traditionally male and female qualities operates to the detriment of both men's and women's health and to the detriment of effective healing. Healing requires a balance between work and love as conveyed through rigorous attention to skill and technique combined with careful sensitivity to, and empathy with, other people and their needs. This book, in part, attempts to redress the balance by drawing attention to the particular importance of connecting effectively with other people in order to promote health and well-being. Following Jean Baker Miller (1986), we want to encourage a greater understanding of growth-enhancing interactions which empower others and, simultaneously, ourselves.

Most practitioners, whether orthodox or complementary in their approach, know that curing disease does not in itself necessarily render the patient healthy. Healing is much more complex than curing: this is a theme which will run throughout the book and to which we will return in the final chapter. We will argue that healing, in its broadest sense of rendering whole, is a social process which takes place through the therapeutic relationship. We follow Cassell (1978) in defining healing as a process of restoring the patient's sense of connectedness, indestructibility and control. An important part of the task of the healer is to relieve suffering, a notion which has been explored in depth by Cassell (1991) in his book *The nature of suffering and the goals of medicine*. We consider the healing process to be the facilitation of those forces for getting better that already exist in the patient and in the patient's social world.

It has been said that, despite their diversity, the common bond which unites the complementary therapies is that 'They all attempt, in varying degrees, to recruit the self-healing capacities of the body' (Fulder 1996: 4). This emphasis on promoting the person's own self-healing is sometimes stated as being in contrast to orthodox medicine's success in challenging disease directly, following scientific diagnosis, with the magic bullets of the drug armamentarium or with surgical techniques. It is disingenuous and simplistic to suggest that current orthodox medicine does not also recognize the significance of the patient's own recuperative powers. All medical systems require a balance between facilitation and intervention; the issue is one of relative emphasis, partly depending on the particular patient and the nature of the disorder being treated. We will explore this further in Chapter 2 on the nature of health and healing. It is the relative emphasis on the patient's participation and self-responsibility along with a highly individualized therapeutic approach which seems to differentiate complementary therapies from biomedicine. Complementary therapies are, by and large, characterized by an emphasis on the person rather than on the disease.

The term 'holistic' is often used to describe the approach of many complementary practitioners. Holism is rarely clearly defined, but it is generally taken to imply a recognition that the whole is more than the sum of the parts: it describes an attempt to consider the whole picture rather than the function of small fragmented aspects in isolation from one another (Stone & Matthews 1996). Holism in health care can be taken to imply three things. First, holism acknowledges that the person's spirit, mind and body interact together to produce an individuality which goes beyond any one single aspect of the self. Thus, holism requires a transcendence of the mind–body split which is implicit in reductionist scientific medicine. Second, holism recognizes that the individual person exists in a context. The physical, social and cultural worlds in which the person lives determine, and in turn are determined by, the nature of the individual's life and experiences. Thus, holism suggests that treatment, or the healing act, is also more than the sum of its component parts. The various aspects of treatment are considered to work together, synergistically creating a complex dynamic system in which each component builds on, and interacts with, the contribution of other components.

The need for a more patient-centred, holistic approach to health care has been much discussed, within both orthodox and complementary medicine. Stewart et al (1995) sympathetically described the growing and competing demands on the doctor for time, availability and commitment and elaborated on how difficult it is to meet patients' expectations given the conflict between commitment to patients' welfare and the need to contain costs. The altruistic concerns of medical practitioners are too often constrained by the limitations of the medical model, as well as by real shortages of time and money and by the shortcomings of health service bureaucracy. Stewart et al suggested that a patient-centred model must include, but go beyond, the conventional biomedical approach to incorporate consideration of the patient as an active participant in treatment. Dr Patrick Pietroni in his book *The greening of medicine* (1991), described the move towards more patient-centred medicine as part of a 'greening process' interpreted as a consequence of various influences in Western society including increased knowledge and information, the growing impact of the self-help and consumer movements, greater awareness of environmental issues and the rise of the 'alternative' medical professions. The common strand is the recognition that life, with its attendant misfortunes and fortunes, including suffering, distress, ill health and healing, only exists and has meaning within a social context.

That orthodox medicine, at its best, certainly does aim to promote those circumstances which allow healing to occur naturally is exemplified in the popular writing of the neurologist Oliver Sacks. In his classic text book on migraine, Sacks (1992) suggested that intense and incessant treatment may serve to aggravate rather than alleviate the malady it seeks to help. A clinic which offered simple treatment (including rest in a darkened room, a pot of tea and a couple of aspirins) produced far more impressive results than anything he had seen in more technically oriented clinics. He speculated that allowing a migraine attack to run its course naturally may lead to a quicker and more satisfying resumption of 'ordinary wellness' than offering treatment which, although aborting the attack, may leave the patient vaguely ill and wretched for a much longer period. He concluded that, in the case of migraine:

... for the vast majority of patients and attacks, the answer does not lie in ever-more-powerful drugs, and medicamental aggressiveness, but a sensitive feeling for suffering, and nature; a deep sense of the healing power of nature itself (*vis medicatrix naturae*), and the humility which seeks to woo nature, but never to bully it. (Sacks 1992: 254)

It is perhaps worth enlarging at this point on Sacks' approach to treatment, since his views are so germane to the theme of this book. He wrote:

The physician must not dominate or be dogmatic to the patient, must not play the expert, insist 'I know best'; he must listen to the patient, listen beneath words; listen to his special, unspoken needs; address his dispositions, the patterns of his life; listen to what his illness, the migraine, is 'saying'. Only then will the path of healing become clear. (Sacks 1992: 255)

This book is focused on the nature of the interaction between the patient and practitioner. We recognize that it is through social and cultural forces that the healing act takes its significance and meaning. Helman (1990) has pulled together evidence about healing in non-Western societies. He documented how folk healing and traditional shamanic approaches place illness in a wider cultural context, by explaining it in familiar terms which reaffirm shared values and by mobilizing social support for the patient, thus maintaining group cohesion and reducing anxiety in the ill person and the family or wider community. In Western medicine, treatment of illness tends to be more individually based, with power vested in the professional status of the expert practitioner whose authority and technical skills provide the leverage for change. The evidence which we will review in Chapter 4 indicates that many people, especially those with chronic or long-term disorders, do wish for the sorts of broad outcomes associated with more collaborative therapeutic relationships, emphasizing their desires for explanation, understanding and care along with a sense of personal control.

Readers who wish to pursue their interest in the anthropological and sociological underpinning of treatment are urged to study the literature on medical anthropology, sociology and social psychology, beginning with Helman's book *Culture, health and illness* (1990), Radley's *Making sense of illness* (1994) and Achterberg et al's book *Rituals of healing* (1994), each of which, from differing perspectives, investigates why healing acts may be effective. Effective healing is said to occur because practitioners are socially validated and because their beliefs and therapeutic activities are significant, meaningful and relevant within their particular culture. In this book, we intend to consider ways in which practitioners, through the therapeutic relationship as practised in Western culture, can meet people's desires for treatment and effectively challenge the symptoms of illness through being meaningful, relevant and respectful of them as individuals within families and social networks.

We will attempt to unravel (in Ch. 3) the complexity of the various components of the act of treatment and then, in Chapter 4, to explore in more detail what is already known about the possible unspoken needs and wants of patients who come for treatment. Although it seems clear that orthodox medicine does, at least in principle, recognize the imperative to recruit the patient's own self-healing, the observation of many patients and practitioners is that modern medicine is actually becoming increasingly technical, while the significance of the healing relationship is, at best, given lip service or, at worst, ignored (Balint et al 1993). There is a risk that overemphasis on technique, along with an increased demand for evidence of clinical effectiveness, may lead complementary practitioners along the same path which splits the patient from the illness and which focuses on curing rather than healing.

An emphasis on the purely technical may lead to fragmentation in health care in many ways, which include:

- a widening rift between patient and practitioner; the practitioner is imbued with power and prestige as the 'owner' of technical expertise, while the patient is seen as the passive recipient whose own knowledge is discounted as irrelevant and who cannot, therefore, take active control of the management of his illness
- dissociation between 'expert' theories (which underpin technical interventions) and patients' own 'lay' theories, leading to mutual misunderstanding and confusion (Tuckett et al 1985)
- separation between diagnosis and treatment for psychological and physical disorders which is unhelpful given the evidence

of considerable overlap between physical and psychological distress (Kat 1994)

• treatment which fragments the person's own experience by focusing on disease (the objective manifestation of disorder which is most amenable to technical interventions), neglecting illness (the person's subjective experience incorporating personal meaning) and de-emphasizing sickness (the social manifestation of illness)

• neglect of those fundamental core themes which can be universally applicable to good consulting and therapeutic encounters.

It seems likely that a recognition of the importance of the therapeutic relationship may help to counteract the tendency for health care to fail to meet individuals' and society's deeper needs. The role of the therapist may be to assist in the establishment of a healthy balance within and between individuals, recognizing the interdependence of genetic endowment, mental, physical and spiritual states and physical and social environment (in Ch. 2 we will consider the notion of health as development). Individual health, growth and development require a setting which is facilitative. The original derivation of the word 'therapist' is from the Greek *therapeutes* (to attend) and the Hippocratic writings describe the role of the therapist as assistant to the natural healing forces.

Chapter 5 is devoted to a consideration of the importance of communication and exploration of the meaning of illness in treatment. The social nature of the process of change in treatment is examined in Chapter 6 while Chapter 7 tackles the difficult question of the use and abuse of power. The central chapter of the book is Chapter 8, in which a model of the treatment process is put forward and its implications explored. Chapter 9 considers the significance of the practitioner's health. Finally, in Chapter 10 we will return to a consideration of the nature of healing to pull together the themes of the book.

WHAT IS DISTINCTIVE ABOUT COMPLEMENTARY MEDICINE?

An emphasis on self-healing gives rise to several distinctive features of complementary treatment which have been summarized by Fulder (1996) and which we will consider here in turn for their implications for the therapeutic relationship.

Distinguishing features of complementary medicine

- Symptoms may only be assessed in relation to a particular person.
- Mental, physical and spiritual aspects of the person may be seen as interdependent.
- A broad definition of health is used.
- There is an emphasis on treating chronic disorders.
- There is a relatively low risk of side-effects.
- The patient is expected to do what he can to help himself.
- There is an emphasis on the patient's perspective.

Symptoms may only be assessed in relation to a particular person

The complementary practitioner aspires to treat the person rather than the disease. The person's difficulties are considered to be only understandable in the context of his constitutional background, life history and current circumstances. Treatment seeks to restore the person to his developmental potential through realigning and restoring imbalances, defects and destructive patterns. Therefore, it is believed to be important to assess both how the impediments to development arose in the first place and what is maintaining the difficulties now. This requires taking a detailed history of the person's past and current experiences. Doing so has significant implications for the therapeutic relationship: telling one's story to someone who is genuinely concerned and interested, who listens, who appreciates its relevance to the person's difficulties can be a profoundly therapeutic experience in itself. Many patients feel that, at last, they and their suffering have been taken seriously.

Mental, physical and spiritual aspects of the person may be seen as interdependent

In complementary therapy, the patient is treated as a whole person, with no barriers between mind, body and spirit. This approach gives him the opportunity to make links between his psychological and physical symptoms, his past and current lifestyle and the issues and events which have been important to him.

Certainly, it is now accepted that physical and psychological distress occur together more frequently than chance alone would allow, and the developing field of psychoneuroimmunology is

providing insights into the mechanisms underlying the relationship between the mind and the body (Martin 1997). It is already
well established that people with more diversified social networks live longer than their counterparts with fewer types of
relationships (House et al 1988) and have less anxiety, depression
and non-specific psychological distress (Cohen & Wills 1985).
Participation in a more diverse social network may influence
motivation to care for oneself by promoting feelings of self-
worth, responsibility, control and meaning in life and it seems
that the impact of these processes on health and illness may be
mediated via the immune system. In terms of both causation and
maintenance of disorder, as well as in recovery, the traditional
distinctions in orthodox medicine between psychiatric disorders,
physical disorders in which a psychological component can be
identified (psychosomatic disorders) and physical disorders without psychological involvement are now outmoded. Rather,
psychosocial factors as well as organic factors may influence the
whole spectrum of health disorders (Steptoe 1991).

A report on the psychological care of medical patients by the
Royal College of Physicians and the Royal College of Psychiatrists
(1995) concluded that modern medicine is orientated towards
technological investigations which may divert attention away
from psychological problems. The bodily expression of psychological distress can lead to costly but unrewarding searches for
organic disease while patients may not be receiving the real help
they need. It was reported that between a quarter and half of all
new medical outpatients experience physical symptoms that
could not be explained on the basis of organic disease alone and
up to half of such patients had underlying anxiety and depression.
Equally, patients who present to orthodox medicine as primarily
psychologically distressed frequently do not receive medical
recognition or care for their bodily disorders. Maguire & Granville-
Grossman (1968) found one-third of consecutive psychiatric
inpatients had significant physical illness which had not been
treated and Hall et al (1980) discovered physical illness requiring
medical treatment in 80% of patients in a US psychiatric assessment centre.

The difficulty for orthodox approaches is that the dualistic
thinking which separates physical from psychological functioning leads to an assumption that illness or symptoms are
either physical or mental, thus leading to the neglect of whatever
is less salient in the person's initial presentation. The advantage

of complementary approaches for the patient is that he can be seen as a whole person whose psychological and physical suffering and distress permeate his whole being. Treatment need not separate out his experiences arbitrarily but, rather, he can be treated in a way which validates his experience of himself as a coherent being.

A broad definition of health is used

The broad view that complementary therapists take of health will be expanded in Chapter 2. An emphasis on the positive aspects of health involves taking seriously, and treating, patients' poor vitality and low resistance. There is a recognition, too, of the significance of convalescence, of the patient gradually building up his reserves of strength and energy after a period of illness. The intention is to help the patient to reach, or regain, a position of optimum well-being so that he is less vulnerable to disease and illness or so that he is better able to cope with chronic conditions which cannot be cured. To do so requires enhancing morale as well as bodily well-being through the therapeutic relationship.

There is an emphasis on treating chronic disorders

Complementary approaches are most at home when dealing with chronic, psychogenic or organic disorders where the patient's own resilience plays a large part in his coping or recovery. This is the area of health care in which orthodox medicine has been less successful. By contrast, orthodox medicine has been strikingly successful in dealing with more acute diseases and injuries, where complementary approaches may have more of an adjunctive role to play. Again, as we will explore, the personal aspects of a positive therapeutic relationship have an essential part to play in promoting resilience.

There is a relatively low risk of negative side-effects

The low incidence of side-effects is often considered to be one of the positive aspects of complementary health care. It is not necessarily always the case that complementary procedures, techniques or remedies are harmless even when practised or prescribed competently; indeed, anything which may have the power to heal may also have the power to harm. However, to the extent that treatment is aimed at self-righting the organism or promoting self-healing as opposed to directly challenging symptoms or diseases, then the risk of direct damage is considered small compared to the risks of more powerfully interventionist treatment.

Nevertheless, Coward (1989) has rightly warned against an assumption that complementary approaches are in some sense 'natural' or, indeed, that naturalness can be equated with harmlessness. It is important to recognize that patients' vulnerability inevitably exposes them to risk of damage as well as the possibility of beneficial change in relation to the practitioner's power, whether that power is personal or technical. We will enlarge on this point in Chapter 8 on the power of the practitioner. For now, it is enough to recognize that the dangers of the abuse of the practitioner's power will be minimized if the patient's own central role in treatment and healing is recognized and strengthened. At the same time, practitioners of all disciplines need to retain an awareness of the limits of their own skills, abilities and knowledge (as well as the limits of the therapies they practise) so that patients are not denied treatment which may be more relevant, appropriate or effective for their needs.

The patient is expected to do what he can to help himself

In most complementary therapies, the patient is seen as an active participant rather than a passive recipient of treatment. This is really quite different from some orthodox health care where patients may be expected to 'comply' with medical treatment but not necessarily to take steps to promote their well-being through changes in lifestyle. Doctors and nurses in orthodox settings often express exasperation that many of their patients, especially those with chronic disorders, do not do enough to help themselves. Indeed, some orthodox practitioners in workshops have expressed envy of complementary practitioners whose patients, almost by definition, are those who have decided to do things differently, take matters into their own hands and who are therefore more likely to be receptive to ideas about taking responsibility for their own health.

In orthodox health care, any inclination the patient may have to take personal responsibility can sometimes be difficult to act on because of the long tradition of authority in medicine, where the doctor has greater technical knowledge and the patient's knowledge may not be viewed as relevant. Moreover, many orthodox doctors feel that the real time constraints in their consultations do not allow them the opportunity to explain and to share information which would motivate the patient to take responsibility for change. The approach in complementary health care makes it easier for practitioners to adopt a more collaborative style with their patients. The aim should be to help the patient to take responsibility for his health, but not to take the blame for his illness. This point will be further elaborated in Chapter 2, where we differentiate between health on the one hand and disease, illness and sickness on the other.

There is an emphasis on the patient's perspective

In this book we want to emphasize the patient's perspective on treatment. For that reason, we have tried to be informed, wherever possible, by patients' stories about their experiences of health care and have chosen not to provide 'case histories' because these tend to oversimplify and trivialize the complexities of real life. We have talked to people who have used complementary treatment, people who have been prepared to share their stories of being on the receiving end of complementary medicine. Both writers have been patients too, as well as psychological practitioners, so we have also drawn on our own personal experiences. Above all, the message of this book is to encourage practitioners to continue, throughout their career, to recognize and respect the wisdom of their patients. Returning again to the words of Oliver Sacks:

There is only one cardinal rule: one must always listen to the patient and, by the same token, the cardinal sin is not listening, ignoring. Prior to any and all specific approaches, there must be this general approach, the establishment of a relation, a communication with the patient, so that patient and physician understand each other. A relationship, moreover, in which the patient is not entirely passive and compliant, believing and doing what he is told, and taking what is 'ordered'; a relationship which is, essentially, collaborative. (Sacks 1992: 252)

REFERENCES

Achterberg J 1990 Woman as healer. Rider, London
Achterberg J, Dossey B, Kolkmeier L 1994 Rituals of healing. Bantam Books, New York
Baker Miller J 1986 Towards a new psychology of women, 2nd edn. Penguin, Harmondsworth
Balint E, Courtney M, Elder A, Hull S, Julian P 1993 The doctor, the patient and the group: Balint revisited. Routledge, London
Brooke E 1993 Women healers through history. Women's Press, London
Cassell E J 1978 The healer's art. Penguin, Harmondsworth
Cassell E J 1991 The nature of suffering and the goals of medicine. Oxford University Press, Oxford
Cohen S, Wills T A 1985 Stress, social support and the buffering hypothesis. Psychological Bulletin 98:310–357
Coward R 1989 The whole truth: the myth of alternative health. Faber and Faber, London
Fulder S 1996 The handbook of complementary medicine. Oxford University Press, Oxford
Hall C W, Gardner E R, Stickney S L, LeCann A F, Popkin M K 1980 Physical illness manifesting as psychiatric disease. Archives of General Psychiatry 37:989–995
Helman C G 1990 Culture, health and illness, 2nd edn. Butterworth Heinemann, Oxford
House J S, Landis K R, Umberson D 1988 Social relationships and health. Science 241:540–545
Kat B 1994 The contribution of psychological knowledge to primary health care: taking a step back to go forward. Clinical Psychology Forum 65:23–26
Maguire G P, Granville-Grossman K L 1968 Physical illness in psychiatric patients. British Journal of Psychiatry 114:1365–1369
Martin P 1997 The sickening mind: brain, behaviour, immunity and disease. HarperCollins, London
Miller J, Bell C 1996 Mapping men's mental health. Journal of Community and Applied Social Psychology 6:317–327
Pietroni P C 1991 The greening of medicine. Gollancz, London
Radley A 1994 Making sense of illness: the social psychology of health and disease. Sage, London
Rowbotham S 1990 Woman's consciousness, man's world. Penguin, Harmondsworth
Royal College of Physicians and Royal College of Psychiatrists 1995 The psychological care of medical patients. Recognition of need and service provision. Royal College of Physicians and the Royal College of Psychiatrists, London
Sacks O 1992 Migraine. Picador, New York
Sanders D 1996 Counselling for psychosomatic problems. Sage, London
Steptoe A 1991 The links between stress and illness. Journal of Psychosomatic Research 35(6):633–644
Stewart M, Brown J B, Weston W W, McWhinney I R, McWilliam C L, Freeman T R 1995 Patient-centred medicine: transforming the clinical method. Sage, London
Stone J, Matthews J 1996 Complementary medicine and the law. Oxford University Press, Oxford
Tuckett D, Boulton M, Olsen C, Williams A 1985 Meetings between experts: an

approach to sharing ideas in medical consultations. Tavistock Publications, London

Ussher J M, Nicolson P 1992 Gender issues in clinical psychology. Routledge, London

Wilkinson R G 1996 Unhealthy societies: the afflictions of inequality. Routledge, London

2

The nature of health and illness

There are two complementary refrains in health care as it has been practised throughout the ages. The first is represented by the myth of Hygeia, whose name originated from the same source as the Greek word for health. She symbolized the belief in health as the natural way of things, that people could remain well if they lived a sane life in a pleasant environment. In this tradition there is an expectation of health as the normal state, which is related to equilibrium and balance, and treatment is seen as a way of aiding the person's own natural, self-healing capacities. The role of the physician is to help the person achieve inner balance (between the physical, emotional and spiritual aspects of themselves) and outer balance (between themselves and their world). The physician's task is to promote health through teaching the natural wisdom by which the person can retain harmony and balance.

The second refrain is represented by the healing god Asclepius, son of Apollo, who is said to have achieved fame through his use of the knife and by knowledge of the curative power of plants. His focus was on dealing with disease, rather than on promoting health. In this tradition, there is an expectation of disorder, disharmony and disease and the role of the physician is to bring external forces to bear to challenge and overcome the disorder in order to bring the individual to an ordered state of health.

These two refrains are represented in the healing traditions by, on the one hand, treatments which emphasize the promotion of the individual's health (usually focused on harnessing the person's own self-healing capacity) and, on the other, treatments which attempt to control and overcome disease and its accompanying symptoms. Ideally, a balanced health care system would incorporate both approaches, shifting the focus when appropriate according to the patient's needs. In practice, it seems that different traditions of health care offer greater strengths in one or the other type of approach: modern Western biomedicine is powerful and effective in the Asclepian tradition of using technical means to fight disorder, while many complementary approaches seem particularly adapted to the Hygeian ideal of promotion of health through balanced living. Similarly, it seems that different disorders may require different emphases: some diseases respond dramatically to technical intervention, while others (especially chronic and degenerative disorders) are less amenable to technique alone and may need broader based approaches in order to influence the course of the illness.

In this chapter we hope to clarify some of the concepts relating on the one hand to health and on the other to disease, illness and sickness. We suggest that health and illness are not opposite ends of one dimension, but rather that they are logically separate, although interconnected, dimensions of a person's being. The terms 'disease', 'illness' and 'sickness' are often used loosely in clinical accounts of treatment, as if they were interchangeable concepts. It is important to draw distinctions to establish precise meanings of these words to help clarify what may be happening in various treatment approaches.

WHAT IS HEALTH?

Positive and negative definitions

The ways in which people define health can be influenced by their sociocultural backgrounds. Health may be defined negatively in terms of the absence of certain negative states or positively in terms of the presence of desired states such as balance, wholeness or energy.

Negative definitions of health involve the absence of disease or bodily abnormality or the feelings of pain or distress that may or may not accompany disease. There are two problems with negative definitions: the first is that they tend to lead to methods of treatment which are focused only on getting rid of symptoms rather than promoting those aspects of living which may be associated with health in a broader sense. The second problem is that negative definitions of health do not, on the whole, accord with ordinary people's views of what is healthy.

A positive definition of health is given in the commonly quoted World Health Organization definition (1946), conveying a sense of health as an 'ideal state': 'Health is a state of complete physical, mental and social well-being and not merely the absence of disease and infirmity'. It seems that many lay beliefs about health have, as their starting point, ideas of the wholeness of human beings. Aggleton (1990) found that people may consider themselves or others healthy irrespective of whether or not they were diseased. What seemed to matter was the wholeness or integrity of the person, their inner strength and their ability to cope. Herzlich (1973), in an interview study of 80 predominantly middle-class people in France, also found that people differentiated between illness on the one hand and health on the other. Illness was seen primarily as something external to the individual, related to pathological agents such as germs and to aspects of the person's lifestyle. Health, on the other hand, was seen as something more intrinsic to the person, determined largely by temperament and heredity. Positive definitions of health were associated with physical strength, resistance to illness and 'equilibrium', described in terms of happiness, relaxation, feeling strong and having good relations with others.

Pill & Stott (1982), in an interview study with mothers from working-class backgrounds, found a commonly used definition of health was having the capacity to function as expected and being able to cope. In his review of lay people's ideas of health, Radley (1994) concluded that health is seen as logically independent of illness, so that it is not simply the opposite of being ill or the condition of someone who has not been given a medical diagnosis.

Instead, concepts of health – as reserve or equilibrium – connect with other areas of life, giving it meaning in terms of feelings and capacities involving activities and other people. (Radley 1994: 41)

In other words, health on the one hand and illness on the other are separate dimensions which do not automatically relate to one another.

Positive definitions of health, in their more theoretical form, can seem idealized and perhaps unrealistic. Dubos (1979), in his book *The mirage of health*, called into question the idea that there could be a state of ideal health. He referred to the illusion which has flourished in many societies, as portrayed, for example, in the Garden of Eden myth, that perfect health and happiness are attainable by humans. In both Eastern and Western philosophies, there has been a notion that at some time in the past there was a period of natural harmony, when man was in perfect accord with his environment and held an internal balance between mind and body.

Any achievement of an ideal state of balance or equilibrium could never last for long, Dubos suggested, since we live in a world in which change is the norm, where the word 'nature' does not designate a definable and constant entity. He considered that there is not one nature but rather only associations of states and circumstances, varying in time and place. Thus, definitions of health which rely on idealized forms of harmony, such as the Tibetan ideal of the balance of the three humours acting as factors to maintain good health (Donden 1986), may imply a rigid, conservative and unattainable approach to health. It is important to note here, however, that the idea of health as a static state is a misrepresentation of the more subtle understanding of the consistency of change, as depicted in many traditional medical systems. Wiseman (1995), for example, in his translation of the ancient texts on fundamental concepts of Chinese medicine, wrote of health being seen as a dynamic harmony and interaction of an inner environment with an exterior world.

Dubos himself emphasized the importance of adaptation to changing circumstances: organisms can only be healthy insofar as they can function and survive in the particular circumstances in which they find themselves. Dubos saw health and happiness as expressions of ways in which individuals respond and adapt to the challenges of everyday life. This idea of health as adaptation is helpful for three reasons.

Benefits of viewing health as adaptation to circumstances

- It is realistic and pragmatic. The view of health as adaptation moves away from what may be seen as an unhealthy yearning and preoccupation with trying to achieve an ideal yet unattainable state of perfect health.
- It accords with lay approaches to health. In everyday terms, people want health not as an end in itself but rather so that they can get on with their lives. Health is something a person can largely take for granted when life is progressing as normal.
- It emphasizes the environment as well as the individual. The idea of health as adaptation leads to the practical implications that the promotion of health requires attention to both the individual *person's* adaptability and to the *environment's* adaptability.

Seedhouse, who reviewed the currently available definitions of health, emphasized the importance of environmental conditions in his definition of health as fulfilment of personal potential: 'A person's health is equivalent to the set of basic conditions which fulfil or enable a person to work to fulfil his or her realistic, chosen and biological potentials' (1986: 72). From this perspective, people can only be healthy if their circumstances and environment are suited to their needs. The challenge here for health care is to find ways to intervene at social and environmental levels to promote communities within which individuals can fulfil their potential.

Health as development

Following Seedhouse, the definition proposed here, emphasizing the individual's own contribution as well as that of the environment, is of health as development. We define health as that state of spiritual, emotional, cognitive, physical, social and environmental functioning which facilitates the individual's development: the balanced, coherent and integrated adjustment of, and accommodation to, internal and external events.

The implication of this definition for health care is that the promotion of health involves finding ways of helping people to continue developing in the face of changing circumstances. There are two aspects to this: adapting to new circumstances through altering established patterns; and acting on the world when possible. The healthy person is both flexible and resilient; able to adapt (within certain limits) yet retaining personal identity. Indeed, development was seen by the psychologist Piaget (1952) as a gradual move towards greater complexity, as a person integrates inner and outer experiences, through assimilating and accommodating to change. Being healthy is thus seen as both responsive and active. From this perspective, insofar as treatment is about promoting health, the task for the practitioner is to facilitate the patient's development.

There is a clear parallel here with the attempt, in all complementary therapies, to recruit the person's own self-healing capacities but there is also an implication that health care may require intervention at social and political levels to ensure an appropriate environment for individual development. Moreover, since development always takes place in a social, interpersonal context, serious attention must be paid to the interpersonal aspects of treatment: that is, the therapeutic relationship. This theme will be further developed in Chapter 7, where we consider the idea of treatment as a developmental process.

DISEASE, ILLNESS AND SICKNESS

When a person becomes unwell, there are (at least) three perspectives of the experience: these focus respectively on the body, the individual's experience and society.

Disease: focus on the body

Here, the concern is with the pathology which may underlie a person's disorder. The concept of disease is very much a phenomenon of modern Western scientific medicine. Clinical signs and symptoms which are observed to occur together can be diagnosed as an entity (disease or syndrome), a 'fact' for which the underlying cause, or chain of causal influences, is sought. The emphasis on objective physiological facts in Western medicine is related to a search for fundamental bodily processes. The notion of 'impairment' is helpful here: the idea that there is something fundamentally wrong with a person's bodily or structural functioning underlies the concept of disease. Helman (1990) described how the task of the doctor in Western medicine is to translate the patient's symptoms to their biological referents in order to discover, or diagnose, the disease entity. This process involves listening to the patient's account of his symptoms and of how the symptoms developed (the history) and then searching for objective physical signs (the examination).

Increasingly, diagnostic technology (scans, blood tests, X-rays, etc.) has led to an emphasis on measurement of bodily functions and to definitions of normality and abnormality through reference to the normal range of the parameter in question (whether it be blood pressure, heart rate, glycaemic level, auditory activity, weight, etc.). The medical definition of disease, therefore, is:

... largely based on objectively demonstrable physical changes in the body's structure or function, which can be quantified by reference to 'normal physiological measurements'. (Helman 1990: 89)

It is the practitioner's perspective which is to the fore when considering disease. It is sometimes said that illness is what patients and their families bring to the practitioner, while disease is what they have after the consultation.

Disease is what the practitioner creates in the recasting of illness in terms of theories of disorder. Disease is what practitioners have been trained to see through the theoretical lenses of their particular form of practice. (Kleinman 1988: 5)

Disease is the problem from the practitioner's perspective: it is what practitioners diagnose and treat.

Illness: the individual's experience

Illness relates to a way of being for the person concerned: how they perceive, appraise and respond to their symptoms, how their lives are affected by the consequences of the symptoms (and the treatment). Illness is a personal, lived experience, dependent not simply on physical or mental impairment but rather on how the impairment manifests itself in the life of a specific individual living in particular circumstances. Illness is what the person feels and experiences.

Aspects of illness

- *Bodily processes*: such as discomfort, pain, nausea, spasms, coughs
- *Mental processes*: including depression and anxiety
- *Relationship issues*: including social isolation, altered sexuality
- *Emotional sequelae*: such as anger, frustration, demoralization, impotence, grief
- *Practical implications*: in terms of daily living, such as inability to dress oneself, walk, go to work, look after children.

The practitioner needs to try to understand the impact of the disorder (and its treatment) on the person's life in physical, mental, social, emotional and practical terms.

Sickness: the social context

The third perspective is that of society: sickness can be understood in two ways.

First, sickness can be seen as the manifestation of disorder at the social level or as the patterning of disease in society. At this level, sickness is seen in relation to the social forces (economic, political and institutional) which maintain the factors (poverty, oppression or envy, and lack of choice) which underpin the distribution of disease in society.

Second, sickness is the particular social role or status accorded to an individual who either experiences illness or who has been diagnosed as having a disease. Parsons (1951a, 1951b) described the process of the adoption of the sick role by which, through the legitimization of the illness by the practitioner, the person is allowed, or required, to remove himself from the demands and expectations of everyday life, while at the same time doing all that he can to cooperate with the physician in getting well again.

There may be conflicting pressures in the potential adoption of the sick role. On the one hand, the sick role may convey some benefits: avoidance of responsibility, continuation of protection and dependence, access to care and attention. In practice, however, there may be a distinct negative side to these putative advantages, especially for those who have long-term sickness. They may be kept in a disadvantaged position without the opportunity to develop social power or choice, without access to economic, material or political resources. Moreover, the care they receive from others may by no means be the loving or encouraging sort of care one would hope to receive.

The sick person may be stigmatized and seen as someone who is other, who is different from healthy people in ways which are judged as inferior. Certain diseases or impairments may be particularly or idiosyncratically stigmatizing, depending upon the prejudices and beliefs about their causes and consequences held in the particular society. AIDS is the obvious example here, but also people with visual impairments, mental health difficulties or physical disabilities have, unfortunately, been stereotyped as passive, insensitive, aggressive or stupid, irrespective of their individual qualities but simply on the basis of the assumed characteristics of their disorder. The person who occupies the sick role is very vulnerable to societal abuse, disempowerment and marginalization.

There is likely to be ambivalence about the sick role: its adoption may convey certain benefits, at least in the short term (and in acute illnesses the benefits of rest, care and abdication of responsibility may be unavoidable as they are thrust on the person by the nature of the symptoms) while long-term occupation of the sick role may in itself impair the person's health through reducing opportunities for development.

THE ROLE OF THE COMPLEMENTARY PRACTITIONER IN DEALING WITH HEALTH, DISEASE, ILLNESS AND SICKNESS

Complementary medicine, at least as practised now in Western society, is most at home in dealing with illness rather than disease or sickness. The usual focus is at the level of the functioning and experience of the individual. In some traditional practices this is placed in the social context, so that ceremonies and rituals may be used to reconnect the individual's life and purpose with that of his tribe or culture, restoring balance to the individual within the moral order of society. However, complementary practitioners rarely intervene at the social level in the West, either because the models they use do not address social issues (as in homeopathy, osteopathy, medical herbalism) or because the theoretical models do not fit with Western culture (as in the case of traditional Chinese medicine or Ayurvedic medicine).

Most complementary practitioners aim to promote health; indeed, we have already seen how Fulder (1996) identified the promotion of self-healing as the common thread which unites the therapies. Again, this is at the level of the individual: while many complementary disciplines have as their foundation approaches to healthy living (involving lifestyle, spirituality, diet, exercise and so on), practitioners have not attempted to implement these at a collective level in an analogous way to orthodox health promotion. It is, of course, possible that in the future complementary and orthodox health care concepts may be integrated into health promotion work, a development awaited with interest. In the meantime, it seems that promoting the health of the individual and dealing with illness is where the complementary practitioner has the greatest contribution to make.

There is a concern in modern medicine now to move beyond the reductionist medical model towards 'holistic' health care. Yet it will be a challenge to integrate alternative models of understanding health and illness with biomedical ideas; the tendency will be for them to be incorporated within biomedicine. In Western society, the biomedical approach is held not to be *an* approach to medicine but rather *the* approach, since it is built on a natural science foundation and deals with 'facts'; biomedical knowledge is held to be objective, neutral and value free. Thus, for example, the oncologist Brewin, chairman of Health Watch, was able to state: 'Mainstream medicine, *since it is not tied to any system or belief*, is free to incorporate any really effective remedy at any time, whether or not its mechanism is understood' (1995: 7) (our italics). This position is in direct contradiction to that of medical anthropologists who, taking a cultural perspective, view the medical system as one domain of cultural knowledge among others and refuse to take the assumptions of any particular system as absolute (Radley 1994).

From the anthropologist's observations, knowledge is not neutral; it also serves the purpose of maintaining one's own view of the world as 'real' and can be exercised to maintain the authority of experts within that knowledge system. The starting point for Western medicine is the treatment of disease; the perspective may have broadened in recent years but diagnosis and effective treatment of disease remain the forte of biomedicine and it is less successful in helping people to deal with the meaning and psychosocial consequences of illness, not least because issues of meaning are considered as secondary to scientific facts.

The systems of belief underlying most complementary medicine do not involve the assumptions of the natural sciences and complementary approaches therefore do not necessarily apply the reductive scientific approach: some may feel that this is at the cost of a relative lack of power, but the benefit is that instead they are required to stay at the level of trying to understand the ill person's experience. Indeed, without a theoretical framework which breaks down understanding into parts, related to organs of the body and classifications of diseases, and without the technology of stethoscope, X-ray machine, surgery, pathology laboratory and so on, the main source of information must remain the patient himself. His story and his symptoms must be central to the practitioner's understanding of the illness.

Kaptchuk (1983) contrasted the analytic approach of Western medicine which starts with a symptom, then searches for the underlying mechanism – a precise cause for a specific disease – with the synthetic approach of Chinese medicine in which the question of cause and effect is secondary to the overall pattern. He said:

Oriental diagnostic technique does not turn up a specific disease entity or a precise cause, but renders an almost poetic, yet workable, description of a whole person. (Kaptchuk 1983: 4)

Complementary practitioners, then, usually claim to treat people rather than to treat diseases. And this (as we will elaborate in Ch. 4) is what patients say they want: they want to have authentic relationships with practitioners who understand them and explain things in ways which make sense and who help to make their illnesses manageable. Patients do also want effective treatments, but not necessarily at the cost of losing their sense of humanity. There is, nevertheless, a pressure to deal with disease: from some patients, from practitioners' own desire to give effective help and from members of the medical establishment who challenge complementary practitioners to demonstrate effectiveness on medical model terms. Patel (1987) and Pietroni (unpublished lecture, 1994) both warned against the dangers of focusing on disease. Patel pointed out that complementary practitioners should take as a warning the increased public discontent with orthodox medicine and be cautious about offering their own promises of cure which, if disappointed, could lead to public disenchantment and a backlash against complementary medicine. Pietroni predicted that in 10 years' time complementary practitioners will be scapegoated if their promises are seen to be unfulfilled.

The strength in complementary medicine lies in taking illness, 'the experience of the patient's suffering in the context of his life story', as the starting point for treatment. The challenge lies in finding that balance between promoting health and tackling the symptoms directly which best suits each individual patient and his particular needs.

REFERENCES

Aggleton P 1990 Health. Routledge, London
Brewin T 1995 What's wrong with alternative medicine? The Skeptic 8(6): 6–9
Donden Y 1986 Health through balance. Snow Lion Publications, New York
Dubos R 1979 The mirage of health. Harper, New York
Fulder S 1996 The handbook of complementary medicine. Oxford University Press, Oxford
Helman C G 1990 Culture, health and illness, 2nd edn. Butterworth Heinemann, Oxford
Herzlich C 1973 Health and illness: a social psychological analysis. Trans. Graham D. Academic Press, London

Kaptchuk T J 1983 The web that has no weaver. Congdon and Weed, New York
Kleinman A 1988 The illness narratives. Basic Books, New York
Parsons T 1951a The social system. Free Press, Glencoe, Illinois
Parsons T 1951b Illness and the role of the physician: a sociological perspective. American Journal of Orthopsychiatry 21:452–460
Patel M S 1987 Evaluation of holistic medicine. Social Science and Medicine 24:169–175
Piaget J 1952 The origins of intelligence in children. International Universities Press, New York
Pill R, Stott N C H 1982 Concepts of illness causation and responsibility: some preliminary data from a sample of working-class mothers. Social Science and Medicine 16:43–52
Radley A 1994 Making sense of illness. Sage, London
Seedhouse D 1986 Health: the foundations for achievement. Wiley, Chichester
Wiseman N (trans) 1995 Fundamentals of Chinese medicine. Paradigm Publications, Brookline, Mass
World Health Organization 1946 Constitution. WHO, Geneva

3

Towards a model of treatment in health care

WHAT HAPPENS IN TREATMENT?

A broad understanding of what happens in clinical healing must take into account the whole range of actions and interactions which take place within a treatment encounter (Coulehan 1987). Many accounts of treatment are written as if the so-called specific, technical or focal aspects of treatment are what really count (the remedy, the manipulation, the drug, the needling), while everything else which happens in the encounter is relegated to the dustbin category of 'placebo factors'. This is primarily due to an emphasis on treating the disease rather than illness or sickness. By adopting tight experimental design in clinical trials, investigators attempt to hold constant everything which impinges on the patient except the supposed active agent (medication or procedure) in order to try to establish a causal relationship between change in the patient and the use of medication or procedure.

As every practitioner knows, in the consulting room things are not so neat or so straightforward. A clinical encounter is enormously complex and may involve the practitioner undertaking a range of diverse activities: conversing with the patient, making a physical examination, giving explanations, offering advice, conveying hope and understanding, as well as prescribing remedies or carrying out procedures. All these exchanges may contribute towards the treatment outcome, where we define outcome in broad terms to include promotion of health as well as improvement in illness, cure of disease and alleviation of sickness. Indeed, it is possible to speculate that the therapeutic relationship, the explanations, the practical advice and the technical interventions may interact and may work most effectively if they are pulled together as a whole in the attempt to facilitate change for the patient. There is a danger that, in focusing too much on technique, the investigator and the practitioner may ignore the importance of the other aspects of treatment and the possibility that they act synergistically, to produce an overall effect which may be different from, or greater than, that of the sum of the parts.

The intention in this chapter is to separate four dimensions of the treatment act, not because in clinical practice they necessarily can or should be separated, but as a step towards building a theoretical framework which can accommodate their significance within treatment as a whole.

TECHNICAL ASPECTS OF TREATMENT: DEALING WITH DISEASE

Technical aspects of treatment are the so-called specific or focal methods by which the practitioner attempts to challenge the patient's symptoms. Techniques may include such disparate actions as prescribing medication, acupuncture needling, massage, manipulation or making psychological interpretations. All involve, to a greater or lesser extent, expert knowledge used to diagnose the patient's problem and to identify which technique is needed and expert skill in the application of the chosen technique.

Buckman & Sabbagh (1993) classified techniques atheoretically, according to their mode of action. They suggested that any technique, in medical traditions throughout the world, will fall into one of the following categories: ingestive, invasive, external, remote or mental. Such a differentiation is merely descriptive; it does not offer any way of understanding why the techniques might be effective.

Techniques can also be differentiated theoretically, through understanding the way in which they relate to the conceptualization of health, disease and illness within any particular medical model or tradition. At the risk of oversimplifying, we offer the following examples. In biomedicine, the use of techniques such as surgery or the prescription of medication is based on an understanding of the biological mechanisms underpinning the disease

---

Mode of action of treatment techniques

- *Ingestive*: where the patient takes in a substance or substances such as foods, drugs, remedies, aromatherapy oils
- *Invasive*: where the patient's body is entered with the use of tools as in surgery, acupuncture needling, vaccination, amniocentesis, forceps deliveries
- *External*: where the patient's body is touched on the outside using particular manipulations such as osteopathic or chiropractic thrusts, massage
- *Remote*: where the patient and practitioner do not necessarily have any kind of direct contact as in some forms of spiritual healing
- *Mental*: where the patient and practitioner communicate to alter the patient's beliefs and ideas, as in the various types of psychotherapy and in some forms of shamanism.

(adapted from Buckman & Sabbagh 1993)

---

processes and the structural or pharmacological effects of drugs or surgery. In dynamic psychotherapy, the technique of interpretation is based on a conceptualization of the unconscious nature of psychological conflict and the emotional effect of insight and expression of feeling. In Chinese acupuncture, the technique of needling depends on understanding the concept of flow of energy, or chi, within the person and the effect of manipulating the chi at certain points along the body in order to balance the subtle energy. In each of these examples, the particular technique used is seen in relation to a theoretical formulation. In some cases, a theoretical model may evolve to explain the observed impact of the technique, or in other cases, a technique may emerge through the application of theory. Sometimes, such as in the use of electroconvulsive therapy in depression, there is no clear theory underpinning the technique.

The application of technique can be described as 'causal treatment' because it assumes that effective treatment results from dealing with the cause of disease. In terms of the differentiation between disease, illness and sickness outlined in the previous chapter, technique can be seen to be focused on tackling disease. Techniques directly challenge the person's symptoms as defined within the particular model used, but do not necessarily deal with the broader aspects of the person's subjective experience within their social world. The use of technique alone may be more effective for disorders whose causal determinants can be clearly identified and less so for those with more complex causes or maintaining factors. This is observed to be the case in practice: specific techniques are especially effective, for example, in dealing with acute diseases with identifiable causes, as seen in the treatment of bacterial infections with penicillin or appendicitis with surgery, and are less effective with chronic and complex multifactorial disorders such as rheumatoid arthritis and other immune system disorders.

The professional has much investment in technique; after all, it is the application of her skills and knowledge in the appropriate technique which differentiates the practitioner from a layperson. The use of technique in medical practice requires the legitimization of professional training and qualifications. There is public outrage when a technique is practised without professional legitimization, however competent the practitioner may be (as in the case, much publicized in the national press in 1995, of an experienced ward sister who successfully removed a patient's appendix under the supervision of a surgeon).

Techniques can be seen to symbolize power in treatment: the power to effect change and the power of the practitioner in relation to the layperson. In many traditions, techniques may also convey in concrete form the apparently magical nature of healing. In Western culture, the power of science, with its attendant technology, has largely superseded the power of magic with its associated ritual and ceremony. The mechanistic rationality of science seems to give rise to a sense of loss of personal significance and meaning for which many people, perhaps increasingly, continue to search. Small wonder, then, that techniques appear so salient in treatment. They are indubitably important, in many cases powerfully effective; they offer hope to the patient and status to the practitioner and yet they are by no means the whole story in any treatment encounter.

THEORETICAL ASPECTS OF TREATMENT. THE FORMULATION OF A STORY: DEALING WITH ILLNESS

The second aspect of the therapeutic act to be considered is the formulation of a 'story' or a theory about the person's illness. One of the important features of a therapeutic encounter is that the patient and the practitioner both try to impose some order or structure onto the experience of illness. People ask: 'Why me?', 'Why now?', 'Why this particular illness?'. The medical anthropologist Kleinman (1988) has argued that people, whether lay or professional, use their own explanatory models through which they structure their understanding of illness around six universal themes, incorporating views about cause, timing, nature, prognosis, consequences and treatment.

Themes within explanatory models of illness

- *Aetiology*: ideas about the cause of illness
- *Time and mode of onset of symptoms*: ideas about the significance of what was happening when the symptoms began
- *Pathology*: ideas about what the illness is and what is going wrong with the person who is ill
- *Course of illness*: ideas about how long the illness might last and how it might develop
- *Consequences of illness*: ideas about the possible effects of the illness on the person's life
- *Treatment*: ideas about what could be done to alleviate or cure the illness.

(adapted from Kleinman 1988)

Patients and practitioners use explanatory models to guide their thinking about how illness may be managed. The content of the ideas held by patient and practitioner, or by practitioners from different traditions, may be very different. Part of the practitioner's task may be to offer the patient her ideas, or formulation, and to combine these with those of the patient. The aim of the therapist who uses cognitive therapy for people who are psychologically distressed is to guide the patient in discovering those 'inaccurate' or 'unhelpful' thoughts and meanings which may be perpetuating the disorder (Beck et al 1979). The terms challenging or reframing can be used for the process whereby the practitioner helps the patient to review his original view of the problem so as to detect any 'inaccuracies', influence feelings and so allow fresh possibilities for action. It is important for the practitioner to try to understand the patient's explanatory model, so that her own formulation can be set in terms which make sense to the patient and acknowledge those parts of the patient's story which are important to him but do not fit easily into her frame of reference.

Dimensions of explanatory models

- *Accuracy*: their correctness according to some criterion of truth
- *Relevance*: the extent to which the salient aspects of the model are significant for the particular illness, in the context of the person's life
- *Utility*: the usefulness of the ideas in the model for helping the patient and practitioner to understand and manage the illness.

Explanatory models of illness may vary according to their accuracy, relevance and utility.

It may be that in practical terms, utility and relevance are at least as important as accuracy. Thus, the biomedical model for a disease, for example diabetes, may be accurate insofar as it correctly identifies the physiological disease processes, useful insofar as it leads to appropriate technical intervention in terms of blood sugar control, yet irrelevant if it ignores the psychological and social difficulties of rigid control of diet and behaviour. However accurate and potentially useful a model may be, it will only be helpful if it accommodates to the circumstances of the person's life in such a way that he can translate its implications into practice. This is why, for example, health education programmes which ignore people's psychological, social and economic circumstances are ineffective in changing some behaviours relating to health, such as diet and smoking. It seems that, in part, biomedical models of illness are unsatisfactory for many patients because they focus primarily on disease processes and less so on the more personal and social meanings of illness.

Kleinman (1988) and Garro (1994) described the way in which patients order their complex experiences of illness – what illness means to them – as personal narratives through which they weave illness experience into the plot of their life stories. They contrasted patients' constructions with the impersonal lifelessness and meaninglessness of the constructs of reductionist science. Sacks, in his account of his own experience as a patient in *A leg to stand on* (1991), conveyed a sense of the importance to the patient of his own story:

There were some difficulties about 'the history' because they wanted to know the 'salient facts' and I wanted to tell them everything, the entire story. Besides, I wasn't quite certain what might or might not be 'salient' in the circumstances. (Sacks 1991: 29)

The medical sociologist Sharma, who undertook an interview study of patients using complementary medicine, emphasized the importance of relevance of the frame of reference provided by the complementary practitioner. She wrote:

To the extent that the practitioner's discourse replaces orthodox explanations with meanings and interpretations which are more satisfactory to the patient, and provides evidence consistent with those meanings, then they may be said to 'work', although not in any clinical sense. (Sharma 1992: 71)

In support of this contention, Sharma reported the joy, relief and delight expressed by some of the patients of complementary practitioners at 'having been offered a new way of looking at their illnesses, that sense of a more relevant order being imposed on problematic experiences' (Sharma 1992: 72). It may be that this possibility of offering a plausible account of chronic or intractable suffering is in part based on the willingness of practitioners to base their formulation on an understanding of the patient's story of his illness and its place in his life. If so, the importance of obtaining a detailed and personally relevant case history, which includes the patient's own formulation, must be emphasized.

Wills (1982) drew attention to the importance of helping patients to make some sort of sense of their problems, while de-emphasizing the idea of truth or accuracy of the model underpinning the story which evolves:

What conceptual frames of reference clients learn, how they integrate new information with their own pre-existing world view, and how basic values and philosophies are communicated in clinical interaction is largely unknown at present. What views of problems are most productive for therapy is a largely unanswered question. But it may not matter greatly what world view is adopted. It may be that any coherent system that provides clients with clear rubrics for understanding their own behaviour, and that of other persons, will introduce into their lives a greater sense of predictability and stability, with a consequent increase in their sense of well-being. (Wills 1982: 396)

PRACTICAL ASPECTS OF TREATMENT. SELF-HELP AND SOCIAL ACTIONS: DEALING WITH SICKNESS

An often understated aspect of treatment, perhaps because it is less professionally challenging and heroic than conceptualizing the illness and applying techniques, is that of offering practical advice about the day-to-day management of illness, so as to promote self-healing to facilitate convalescence and to prevent future recurrence.

The anthropologist Helman (1978), in his well-known article 'Feed a cold; starve a fever', demonstrated how, at a folk level, people share with one another their ideas and beliefs about how to manage common illnesses. Traditionally, ideas about what to do when ill are generated through lay beliefs about illnesses which are communicated between the extended family and the wider community. However, when such networks break down, people are left without recourse to traditional sources of advice and are increasingly likely to turn to experts for ideas about what they should do in order to help themselves. In biomedical encounters, this practical advice is often not forthcoming when the focus of the encounter is mainly about diagnosis and treatment. Patients may feel dissatisfied: for example, a parent who took a child with a hacking cough to the GP said 'He didn't give me a prescription and he didn't tell me what to do'. Not knowing whether to send the child to school, keep him in bed, keep him warm or cool, give him particular food or drinks, the mother was left feeling helpless and incompetent. Marsh (1977) noted that when GPs changed their practice to reduce the number of prescriptions for 'minor' complaints, they seemed to balance this by giving more practical advice.

As we will find in Chapter 4, patients want to know whether they can play a part in managing their illnesses and what they can do (if anything) in practical terms to reduce the impact of illness and of the treatment on their lives. Practical advice and access to information are necessary to help the patient regain a sense of control and mastery over the illness. It is also important in terms of assuaging guilt: if there is nothing further that the patient could do, he needs to be convinced of this, so that he is not left with the nagging doubt of 'If only I had...'.

Giving guidance about practical self-help strategies forms that part of the treatment encounter in which the practitioner deals with sickness: that is, dealing with the consequences of illness in the social world. Ideas for practical action may include ways of coping with or managing the outside world: whether and for how long to stay home from work (perhaps including the issue of a 'sick note') or finding outside agencies who may offer help (for example, involving social services, self-help groups, voluntary agencies). Other strategies may depend on the patient's social and family network: gaining support and care during periods of increased dependency balanced with encouragement of independent activity when possible. Practical advice may relate more directly to the person's own management of their life: sleep, rest, exercise, nutrition and diet, sexual activity, control of the immediate environment (such as light, warmth or noise). In order for treatment as a whole to be coherent, relevant and maximally beneficial for the patient, attention to these practical aspects needs to be integrated into the clinical encounter.

Attention to the patient's sickness may require redirecting the focus of treatment to the family or even the community. Various writers, including social anthropologists, feminist clinicians, family therapists and those working in the disability movement, have drawn attention to the importance of focusing on patterns of communications and power relationships within the social environment as a way of understanding the significance and meaning of suffering, of facilitating the possibility of change for individual sufferers and of preventing illness within the community. Scheper-Hughes (1991), writing from the perspective of Chinese medicine, proposed that much stress and suffering can be understood as an expression of social oppression. Illness and the assumption of the sick role can, at times, be an act of defiance which expresses itself in various ways, such as a refusal to work or to struggle under oppressive and self-defeating conditions or as an inability to endure and cope with what is not endurable. Part of dealing with sickness can involve an acknowledgement of individual limitations in dealing with suffering brought about by injustice and inequalities.

RELATIONSHIP ASPECTS OF TREATMENT: DEALING WITH THE ILL PERSON

At the heart of any treatment encounter is the therapeutic relationship between the practitioner and patient. This is central to treatment for two related reasons: first, because it is through the relationship that the patient may be persuaded to take on board the practitioner's method of help; and second, because the experience of being cared for within the therapeutic relationship contributes to healing in itself. The help offered by the practitioner (the specific techniques, the understanding of the illness and the practical advice) can only be useful to the patient if he agrees, at some level, to accept the treatment. The therapeutic relationship (the trust, realistic hope and confidence which the practitioner can inspire in the patient) is the means by which the patient may be persuaded to engage with treatment. Kleinman wrote that:

The chief sources of therapeutic efficacy are the development of a successful therapeutic relationship and the rhetorical use of the practitioner's personality and communicative skills to empower the patient and persuade him towards more successful coping. (Kleinman 1988: 247)

It is as if the practitioner uses herself as the lever to move the patient towards change.

Jerome Frank, in his book *Persuasion and healing* (1973), considered therapeutic methods to be approaches to persuasion. He described the way in which ill people become demoralized: in terms of the psychological aspects of the illness, they lose confidence, they do not feel capable of dealing with further aspects of their lives and they may experience shame, guilt and helplessness. Even if they perceive that there are things they could do to improve their situation, they do not believe they are capable of doing these things. Because of the physical aspects of the illness, they lose the capacity and energy to manage their own lives. There is a relief, for the patient, in finding someone who will join with him in the struggle and to whom he can, at least for the time being, ascribe the power of commanding the resources to help. The aim of therapy, then, is to support the patient and to provide him with morale-enhancing experiences, until he regains his own strength. The patient is persuaded to use the practitioner's resources through the therapeutic relationship, including trust in the therapist, expectation of positive results, emotional commitment to the therapeutic procedure and experience of the therapist's warmth, authority and care.

It is the experience of care which leads on to the second reason for the importance of the therapeutic relationship. Having a relationship with someone significant who cares enough to use her power on the patient's behalf can, in and of itself, bring relief to the suffering patient. It is important to be listened to as someone who matters and whose story is significant and to be treated as someone whose life and troubles are worth attending to in a serious and respectful way. If this happens, then the patient can feel trust in the practitioner and can be convinced of his own worth. Being found worthy of the help offered by someone whom he trusts and respects may lead the patient to regain faith in himself, thus mobilizing his own self-healing resources. Treatment, or healing, should help the patient to 'feel better in himself' even in chronic or life-threatening illness which cannot be 'cured'. This is why love for the patient is central to healing (Lomas 1987) and the most important 'drug' in treatment is the personality of the doctor (Balint 1964).

SUMMARY

We can summarize the main themes of this chapter under four headings: techniques, theory, practical action and the therapeutic relationship.

Techniques

Techniques are important both directly and symbolically. Their appropriate use can lead directly to physical and/or psychological change, especially where there are clear causal determinants for symptoms. The relevance and significance of techniques derive from their link with the practitioner's theoretical framework: in part, the techniques work because it makes sense that they should work. Technique and theory should fit together to provide a believable and convincing rationale for treatment. Techniques symbolize the power of treatment and of the practitioner.

Theory

Theory provides the framework through which the practitioner tries to order and make sense of the patient's illness. The practitioner's use of technique and her advice about practical action will be structured through the application of her own theoretical model to the particular illness and story presented by the patient. The patient also has a theory about his illness which may or may not coincide with that of the practitioner. The practitioner needs to try to understand the patient's theory (explanatory model) so that she can present her story, and her actions which stem from it, in a way which is relevant for the patient's understanding and his life circumstances.

Practical action

Practical action provides the means by which the practitioner can empower the patient, to help him towards understanding what he can do to cope with his illness. Attention to the patient's own possibilities for action and self-care provide a balance in treatment away from dependency, or professional powerful control, towards enhancing the patient's own sense of personal power and self-efficacy.

The therapeutic relationship

The relationship between patient and practitioner lies at the heart of the therapeutic encounter: the practitioner must convince the patient that she cares about him, must listen to the patient's story, must imaginatively put herself in the patient's situation to understand what he feels and must be sensitive to his needs as he changes over the course of treatment. Yet this is not enough: the practitioner must also believe in the effectiveness of the techniques she offers, in her own understanding of illness and in her

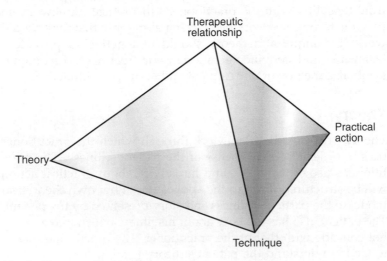

Fig. 1   The pyramid of healing.

own effectiveness as a person. She must believe in the whole treatment she offers in order to convince the patient to persist and not to give up hope. She must persuade the patient towards health.

THE TREATMENT ACT: A MODEL

Based on a consideration of all the aspects of treatment outlined so far in this chapter, we can now propose a model of treatment with four components, which may interact together in order to be maximally effective. They are shown diagrammatically in the form of a three-sided pyramid, described as the pyramid of healing (Fig. 1).

The pyramid of healing

- *Base* (theory, technique and practical action): impersonal treatment, such as might be encountered in surgery or any application of technique or giving of advice where no relationship is established between practitioner and patient
- *Left face* (theory, technique and therapeutic relationship): acute health care, where the patient is too unwell to engage in self-help activity
- *Right face* (therapeutic relationship, technique and practical action): the most basic aspects of healing, such as making the patient comfortable, giving first aid or responding to the patient's needs, much of which is incorporated in good nursing care
- *Back face* (therapeutic relationship, theory and practical action): health promotion and convalescent care.

Treatment seen as a whole requires balance: balance between the personal and the technical, between the art and the craft, between the expert and the lay approaches, between understanding and doing. The pyramid of healing symbolizes the triangle of theory, technique and practical action pulled together to make a solid whole by the therapeutic relationship.

REFERENCES

Balint M 1964 The doctor, his patient and the illness, 2nd edn. Pitman Medical, London
Beck A T, Rush A J, Shaw B F, Emery G 1979 Cognitive therapy of depression. Guilford, New York

Buckman R, Sabbagh K 1993 Magical medicine: an investigation of healing and healers. Prometheus Books, Amhurst
Coulehan J L 1987 The treatment act: a model with focal, behavioral and symbolic dimensions. In: Wilkinson D Y, Sussman M B (eds) Alternative health maintenance and healing for families. Haworth Press, New York
Frank J 1973 Persuasion and healing, 2nd edn. Johns Hopkins University Press, Baltimore
Garro L C 1994 Narrative representations of chronic illness experience: cultural models of illness, mind and body in stories concerning the temporomandibular joint. Social Science and Medicine 38(6):775–788
Helman C G 1978 'Feed a cold, starve a fever.' Folk models of infection in an English suburban community and their relation to medical treatment. Culture, Medicine and Psychiatry 2:107–137
Kleinman A 1988 The illness narratives. Basic Books, New York
Lomas P 1987 The limits of interpretation. Penguin, Harmondsworth
Marsh G N 1977 'Curing' minor illness in general practice. British Medical Journal 2:1267–1269
Sacks O 1991 A leg to stand on, revised edn. Picador, London
Scheper-Hughes N 1991 The rebel body: the subversive meanings of illness. Traditional Acupuncture Society Journal 10:3–10
Sharma U 1992 Complementary medicine today: practitioners and patients. Routledge, London
Wills T A 1982 Non-specific factors in helping relationships. In: Wills T A (ed) Basic processes in helping relationships. Academic Press, New York, ch 17, p 381

4

What do patients want?

The purpose of this chapter is to help to make us more aware of the range of outcomes which any one individual may be hoping for when he consults a health care practitioner. As practitioners, when faced with a particular patient, it is important not to assume that we know what the patient wants. The most usual assumption is that the patient comes for treatment because he wants relief from his symptoms yet, as we will see below, it seems that while many patients do indeed want this, many want more or other things as well.

It is surprising how little attention has been paid, until relatively recently, to trying to find out systematically what patients really want. In an editorial in *Social Science and Medicine*, Mooney (1994) drew attention to the curious convention of *not* asking patients or citizens what they want from health services. To the extent that health service provision has been professionalized, the values and assumptions that prevail are those of the professionals or, as George Bernard Shaw put it more succinctly in *The doctor's dilemma*, '... all professions are a conspiracy against the laity'. It requires a major effort to discern the views of the layperson amongst all that is written on what health care ought to be about. The dominance of professionals' assumptions (the relative power of the professionals) may make it difficult for patients to conceptualize, let alone articulate, that what they want from health care may not always be what the professional seems to be offering. Despite this background belief that 'the doctor knows best', there has been, since the early 1960s, a growing willingness amongst laypeople to question medical authority. This has been documented, for example, by

Cartwright & Anderson (1981) in their follow-up study of patients' views about general practice. They found that, compared with their previous study in the 1960s, patients were becoming more knowledgeable about health matters, more self-confident, less passively accepting and more suspicious of and reluctant to take drugs.

One of the more radical and exciting sources of patients' own views is the user participation and advocacy movement in which people are finding it easier to speak up about their concerns if they have the support of others who share their perspective. This movement represents the desire of people to have a real voice in health care and to have more say and control over their own lives. This work is largely emerging through people with long-term health care needs who have frequently felt marginalized and disempowered. Since patients with chronic conditions form the bulk of those coming for complementary health care (Fulder 1996, Sharma 1992), their point of view as expressed through the patient participation movement warrants serious consideration here. The sorts of views being expressed are demonstrated by Croft & Beresford (1993) in a practical manual for user involvement which emphasizes people's desires: to be treated as real people, with real feelings; to be involved with planning decisions at a policy level as well as an individual level; to be given full access to information; to work in partnership with professionals.

Part of the emphasis coming from the user participation movement is focused on a desire to alter the human values underpinning health care provision. This emphasis on values is often implicit rather than explicit. For example, Annie Mitchell facilitated an advisory panel of people who use, or care for people who use, long-term community health care services. The task was to comment on the training of managers in health and social services. Consultation with various groups of similar people (over 200 people in all) revealed a wide consensus of concern about the apparent overemphasis on efficiency and financial considerations along with a relative neglect of human values. People felt that service provision as represented through managers' preoccupations, often seemed anonymous, detached, hard to pin down, remote from awareness of people's everyday lives and concerns and unduly emphasizing efficiency to the detriment of care for the individual person. The patients' own emphases were on collaborative therapeutic partnerships, mutual respect and understanding and 'tender loving care'. They saw systems and rules currently having priority over personal relationships and they wanted the balance to be tipped the other way. The advisory group concluded that the priority in health care should be to establish caring relationships, characterized by good two-way communication and a mutual respect and recognition of the differing expertise, skills and knowledge held by patients as well as professionals (Consumer Advisory Panel, 1997).

It has been argued elsewhere (Mitchell, unpublished paper, 1994) that patients are asking for a different ethical framework; a shift away from the prevailing ethic of *justice*, predicated on an emphasis on individuality and characterized by objectivity and impartiality, towards an ethic of *care* predicated on an emphasis on relationships, with attention to questions of subjectivity and partiality (see Gilligan (1982) and Gilligan et al (1988) for an introduction to these differing ethical perspectives). Sang (unpublished paper, 1995), who has worked in the advocacy movement for many years, has called for an 'ethic of principled practice': a need for practitioners to engage in a dialogue with patients or service users so that they can apply a knowledge of the individual concerns of patients to their understanding of the general issues involved. This requires a reversal of the usual application of the general to the particular, which is the basis of the reductionist scientific model. The requirement is to begin with the needs and wants of the particular individual with whom the practitioner is faced, rather than trying to fit the individual into general laws and patterns: an approach which sits comfortably with the underlying philosophy of much of complementary health care, as outlined in Chapter 1.

There have recently been attempts by professionals to find out, through systematic evaluation, what people want from their health care. The evidence demonstrates that patients do have a broader agenda than just effective treatment of narrowly defined disease. Indeed, patients' concerns and desires map onto the sort of broad conceptualization of health care set out in Chapter 3, incorporating the four aspects of treatment: techniques; therapeutic relationship; explanation and understanding; practical action and self-help activities.

RESEARCH ON PATIENTS' VIEWS OF TREATMENT

McIver (1993) summarized the cumulative findings of research into patients' views and identified the core themes which seem to be of concern to patients whichever service they are using.

Core concerns of patients

- Effective treatment and care
- Relationships with health care professionals based on good communication and being treated as a person
- Good information to help allay anxiety
- A feeling of control.

Let us consider each of these themes in turn, looking first at the evidence about what patients want (from orthodox and complementary health care) and then considering the implications for practice.

Effective treatment and cure

There is some evidence that patients and professionals may apply different criteria to judge what is effective treatment: clinicians tend to place more stress on physical outcomes, whereas for patients the psychosocial outcome may be equally relevant (Coulter 1994).

Increasingly, patients are inclined to balance the potential benefits of treatment against its costs, in terms of both impact on their quality of life and long-term side-effects of medication or surgery. It is generally considered that the more acute, severe and immediately life-threatening the illness, the higher the priority the patient will place on the technical, probably physical, outcome of treatment. If about to die of appendicitis, for example, most people will consider the risks and discomfort of surgery, which will almost certainly save your life, to be a price worth paying. However, for many illnesses the equation is far from clear. Take the management of diabetes, already mentioned in Chapter 3: for the clinician, glycaemic control is often seen as the priority, apparently reasonably enough given that good control delays the onset and progression of further complication. Yet for many patients, in practice, the restriction on ordinary living imposed by the demanding regime may not be worth the symptom control thus gained (Sowden et al 1995). Patients actively weigh up the costs and benefits of treatment in their own terms.

Some investigators of the use of complementary treatments have emphasized patients' pragmatism in searching for cures or symptom control in conditions which have proved intractable to orthodox treatment (Sharma 1992). The initial motivation in seeking complementary medical help is seen to be a straight-forward need to cure a particular health problem, on terms which the patient accepts. For many patients, cure or treatment of symptoms will be their first priority. Some studies have indicated, however, that for other patients cure or symptom control are not necessarily their highest priority. In an interview study with 20 patients who used complementary treatment, Murray & Shepherd (1993) found that questions of efficacy and scientific research were regarded as secondary to the patients' desires to avoid any possible long-term dangers from modern medical interventions. This was especially the case for treatment of common childhood illnesses such as infantile eczema, recurrent ear infections and tonsillitis. There is the suggestion here, then, that for at least some chronic conditions, patients may prefer the less invasive treatments offered by complementary health care, even if they prove to be less effective in changing symptoms than orthodox treatments.

In a small open-ended questionnaire study (Mills, unpublished work, 1997), patients were asked to write in their own words what they hoped for in treatment (before their first encounter with a complementary practitioner). Of the 50 patients who returned their questionnaires, most did say that they hoped for a cure or improvement. The other themes which emerged were that people were looking for: hope, reassurance, encouragement and understanding, to be listened to, explanation and infor-mation about their conditions, advice about looking after them-selves. One patient who was suffering from hypertension and who felt frightened, powerless, often tense, tired and depressed, put the hope for cure or improvement into context in his answer to the question 'What would you like the practitioner to do for you?':

Cure me – an improvement would be acceptable and I would therefore feel more optimistic about curing myself. My full participation in my treatment as well as information is of the utmost importance.

It is often suggested that patients with terminal illnesses come for complementary health care in the hope of finding a miracle cure. This may indeed sometimes be the case or even always be the case at some level: we may all hope to defy death if only we could. However, recent evidence from patients with AIDS (Langewitz et al 1994) and cancer (Stevenson 1995) who use complementary health treatment does not fully support this idea of a search for miracle cures.

Anderson et al (1993), in a questionnaire study of HIV-positive patients, found that 40% of patients had used alternative therapies. Of those who indicated their expectations, 21% cited 'cure' as one of the results expected from the therapy, whereas half of the sample hoped, more realistically, for delay in onset of symptoms and better immunity. Hand (1989) interviewed 50 patients with AIDS, of whom 18 were using one or more alternative therapies. All the patients with AIDS who used alternative treatments thought they were of value, but none expected the treatment to be curative.

In a questionnaire study of 120 in- and outpatients attending the Royal London Homeopathic Hospital for complementary cancer treatments, Stevenson (1995) asked patients to identify the symptoms for which they would like help from complementary therapies. People most frequently mentioned that they were looking for help with psychological symptoms such as stress and anxiety, whereas help for problems of a physical nature emerged as a much lower priority. This emphasis on the potential mental, as well as physical, benefits of complementary treatment was also found in a questionnaire study of cancer patients who were primarily receiving orthodox care (Downer et al 1994). Sixteen percent of respondents had used complementary treatment in addition to orthodox approaches and they reported high satisfaction with the complementary care they received, which gave benefits including feeling calmer, emotionally stronger, more able to cope with the demands of the illness, more optimistic and hopeful, less difficulty in breathing, increased energy and reduced nausea. When asked to explain their attraction to complementary therapy, people said (in order of frequency of response): they felt more hopeful than when using conventional treatment alone; they were attracted to the perceived non-toxic, holistic nature of the remedies; they wanted more patient participation in treatment; the supportive relationship with the practitioner was important.

Further research on why patients turn to complementary medicine (Vincent & Furnham 1996) confirms Sharma's observation that although patients may initially seek alternative treatment, at least in part because of the ineffectiveness of orthodox treatment for their particular complaints, they also appreciate the particular qualities of complementary approaches. It seems that patients are initially searching for more effective treatment, but in continuing to use complementary approaches (often alongside orthodox health care), other factors become more important. In particular, patients say that they value an emphasis on treating the whole person. Vincent & Furnham (1996) noted the limited research in this area: future studies need to separate the reasons for beginning complementary treatment from those for continuing to use it.

Implications for practice

There are two important implications for practice when considering the issue of effective treatment and cure. The first is that when treatment is clearly aimed at trying to treat or cure particular symptoms, complementary practitioners have the same responsibility as any other health care practitioner: to evaluate systematically their treatments for effectiveness and to apply their techniques rigorously, responsibly and carefully. The second is to be aware that patients are not necessarily only coming to complementary health care directly for relief of symptoms. It is in everyone's interests to be realistic about what can be offered in treatment and to see cure and symptom reduction as only part of the overall picture.

Therapeutic relationship

Over and over again, in studies of patients' views and impressions of treatment, patients say that they care very much indeed about how they are treated as people by health care practitioners. The research on counselling and psychotherapy demonstrates that it may be the experience of the therapeutic relationship *in itself* which facilitates change. Howe (1993) summarized the published evidence about what clients of psychotherapists and counsellors value about how they are treated. He identified the following themes: comfort; the therapist being a real person; the relationship; truth and honesty; support and being there.

What patients value in counselling

- *Comfort*: people want ordinary, human friendliness and warmth. They do not like to be treated blankly, with neutral objectivity.
- *The therapist being a real person*: people like to feel that the therapist is a genuine, straightforward, real person with whom they can engage, someone who is at ease with her own personality but who does not impose or invade the patient with her own views or self-revelations.
- *The relationship*: people value the experience of a therapeutic relationship with a real person who gives comfort, who cares and who provides safety for the exploration of difficult feelings. People appreciate the sense that they themselves matter to the practitioner. In some cases, this can be a long-term feeling, even when there is no sustained contact between the client and practitioner.
- *Truth and honesty*: clients require therapists to be honest and open so that they can know where they stand and so that they can develop a sense of mutual trust.
- *Support and being there*: clients derive a great deal of help from knowing that there is someone available who cares about them and who can provide help and comfort when needed.

(adapted from Howe 1993)

In summary, patients themselves value therapeutic relationships which offer respect, trust and care and it seems that such relationships may in themselves prove to be healing in the broadest sense.

The main theme which emerges from the research on patient satisfaction in orthodox health care is the high priority which patients put on how health care is delivered, especially the way in which they are treated by those who offer the care. In a literature review of patient views on quality of care in general practice, Rees-Lewis (1994) concluded that the factor which is most consistently identified as being of particular value to patients is interpersonal skill on the part of the practitioner.

There is reason for supposing that patients of complementary practitioners see the therapeutic relationship as central to the consultation and that many have become dissatisfied with their relationships with orthodox practitioners. Cassileth et al (1984) found that cancer patients who sought alternative treatment were less likely to perceive their relationship with their physician as good than were those who did not seek out alternative treatment. In the detailed interview study of 20 patients mentioned earlier, Murray & Shepherd (1993) found that the therapist's time and attention were the aspects of alternative medicine most highly valued by patients. Even when the reported experiences of alternative medicine had not been entirely favourable, people maintained positive attitudes towards the alternative care, 'mainly because expectations of cure were secondary to the interest shown by practitioners in the patients' views of their problems' (p. 987). People appreciate the time which alternative practitioners can usually devote to the individual patient, in contrast to the time limitations within National Health Service (NHS) practice.

Patients recognize, though, that it is not simply a matter of time, but that orthodox medical training, with its emphasis on scientific rationality, may act as a constraint on doctors' valuing the human, personal aspects of the consultation. Shifrin (1995) noted the possibility of the imposition of too much rationality within complementary health care, warning that the increasing emphasis on the measurement of tangible outcomes should not occur at the expense of less tangible qualities, such as integrity, humanity, caring and confidentiality, since it may be the loss of some of these qualities amongst doctors that has led to the move towards complementary medicine.

Implications for practice

The implication of the importance placed by patients on the therapeutic relationship is clear: practitioners need to use their own personal qualities to try to establish safe, respectful and reliable therapeutic relationships in which they offer comfort and care to their patients. The significance of the therapeutic relationship should be taught both in the initial training of complementary practitioners and in postqualification supervision and training.

Information

One aspect of the therapeutic relationship which matters very much to patients is the practitioner's ability and willingness to communicate effectively, both in terms of finding out what is important from the patient's point of view and in conveying information and explanations back to the patient. The issue of doctor–patient communication has been systematically reviewed by Ley (1988) who concluded that the majority of patients wish to know as much as possible about their illness, its causes, its treatment and its outcome. In orthodox health care, it has been found that the giving of information by GPs is one of the best predictors of patient satisfaction (Steptoe 1991). At the same time, there is much evidence that there are often problems in doctor–patient communication and that patients are frequently critical of the extent to which doctors give explanations to patients (Cartwright 1967, Cartwright & Anderson 1981). Some of the issues and difficulties about achieving a shared dialogue between patients and doctors will be expanded in Chapter 5. Good information helps to allay anxiety and can give a feeling of control which may have a direct association with the achievement of better outcomes. McIver (1993) reviewed a number of studies and concluded that better outcomes were achieved when patients had received more information, had had more opportunity to express emotion and had been more able to exercise control in the consultation.

As already discussed in Chapter 3, patients come to consultations with their own ideas, questions, fears and worries about what might be wrong with them, what could be done and what the future might hold. From the patient's perspective an important purpose of the consultation is to check out these ideas: 'What has caused the illness? What can be done about it by myself as well as by the practitioner?' For many patients, having a conversation with the practitioner about such questions may be important as an end in itself, as well as a means towards achieving a more satisfactory outcome in terms of managing the illness. The well-documented difficulties for patients in establishing this sort of dialogue in orthodox health care (Tuckett et al 1985) demonstrate the importance of communicating openly and respectfully.

Implications for practice

Recognizing the importance of providing relevant information in practice means paying attention to and being explicit about the patient's and the practitioner's beliefs, questions and knowledge about illness and treatment. It is important at the outset to clarify what the patient already knows and believes (or the questions he has) about his illness. At the end of the consultation, it can be helpful to summarize the practitioner's views, setting them out explicitly so as to help the patient make sense of any treatment which is offered, under headings such as the following.

- *This is what I think is the matter . . .*
- *This is what I think about why this may have happened to you . . .*
- *This is the treatment I can offer . . .*
- *and this is why I think the treatment will help . . .*
- *You may notice these side-effects . . .*
- *and these benefits . . .*
- *This is what you can do to help yourself . . .*
- *Come back to see me when or if . . .*
- *Is there anything more you would like to check with me?*

Control within treatment

The desire for more patient participation in treatment is a constant theme in the literature on patients' perspectives on health care (e.g. Cartwright & Anderson 1981). There is, by and large, a desire for more egalitarian relationships between laypeople and health care providers which is embodied in the new consumerism. A cursory glance at the health section of any bookshop shows the extent of the burgeoning literature on self-help in health care. Many people want to know what they can do to help themselves and those they are caring for when they are ill.

The complicated relationship between patients' understandings and beliefs about illness and treatment, the desire for relevant information and the need to feel a sense of control has been exemplified in a qualitative study looking at the concerns of parents when their preschool children are acutely ill (Kai 1996). The parents of 95 preschool children in a disadvantaged inner city area were interviewed about coping with acute illness in their children. Many thought that they did not get enough information or explanation from their GP when the child was ill: a simple label of virus or bug was unsatisfactory because it seemed too vague and did not offer a sense of being in control or of what they should look out for and do in order to manage the illness. One mother said: 'It's the not knowing what it could be – how to tell – that's what panics me. If I was told what to do, shown what to do and how to do it, I would feel I could manage much better' (Kai 1996: 989). Kai himself concluded:

Professionals have considerable potential to empower parents by sharing more information and skills. Such information should be consistent and address parents' concerns, beliefs and expressed needs if this potential is to be realized. (Kai 1996: 987)

Research on the views of people who use mental health services provides strong evidence of the value users place on approaches which promote personal coping (Mitchell in press). In a survey of over 400 people's experiences of mental health services and treatments (Mental Health Foundation 1997), it was found that people in emotional distress used a variety of methods to attempt to take control of their lives. They developed their own individual ways of coping, which brought a whole range of everyday activities, therapies and treatments into an overall strategy for living with mental health problems. Users expressed strong appreciation for 'talking treatments' (counselling and psychotherapy) and for a range of alternative and complementary therapies, finding them much more helpful than psychiatric approaches (medication with antidepressants or major tranquillizers or electroconvulsive therapy). Nearly half of the people surveyed had experienced art or creative therapies, reporting benefits such as expressing feelings, focusing the mind, distraction, relaxation, support and receiving empathy. One-third had tried physical therapies, including osteopathy, aromatherapy, acupuncture, massage and reflexology, and exercise and postural therapies, such as yoga, Alexander technique and physical exercise. Various benefits were mentioned, in particular relaxation, being treated as a whole person and taking greater control of their own treatment. Naturopathy, herbalism and homeopathy had been tried by a quarter of those surveyed, with more equivocal benefits. These approaches involved a more passive acceptance of treatment, possibly leading to similar expectations to those promoted by conventional medical treatment. The positive benefits of complementary therapies could be summarized as promoting a sense of structure and meaning in life, similar to the effects of hobbies, leisure activities and spiritual support.

It would seem that part of the attraction of complementary approaches lies in the potential for helping people to look after themselves more effectively through giving guidance on lifestyle issues. A quote from the previously mentioned study of complementary patients (Mills, unpublished work, 1997) illustrate the importance of participation and control in treatment. In answer to the question 'What are you expecting from your treatment?' one person wrote:

I would like to know what is going on. If I know what it is and how it is likely to respond to treatment – or not (it might mean a change in diet) – I can then make choices. I feel that if I understand it I have more control. The practitioner may even be able to sort it out for good by prescribing something, but that is not my first priority. I want to know exactly what it is and why it is happening, or why it occurred.

Sharma (1992) noted how people who used non-orthodox medicine were apt to express a sense of greater control over their lives as a result and described immense satisfaction in this new self-reliance. One interviewee commented: 'I make up my own mind about these things. Before, I just accepted it (the discomfort of chronic rhinitis). Now I feel I am in control of my life' (Sharma 1992: 51).

Implications for practice: the need for patient–practitioner collaboration

Three strands emerge in considering the issue of control of treatment. First, there is a sense in which control comes through knowledge and information. As noted in the previous section, patients feel more in control when they understand what is going on and when they feel that they have been understood by the practitioner. Second, a sense of control emerges through the sharing of power within the therapeutic relationship. This issue of power in therapy is explored in Chapter 7. Third, control comes through being able to do something oneself in order to manage the illness. This is where the practitioner can help in concrete, tangible ways through linking explanations to advice. A word of caution is in order here. Although many patients *do* want the sense of control that goes with taking action to help themselves, this will not be the case for everyone and may depend on the acuteness, severity and stage of the illness. Moreover, patients should not be burdened with excessive responsibility for their own well-being. Therapeutic zeal and optimism must be tempered with a recognition of real constraints and limitations.

SUMMARY

From the patient's point of view, there are a range of possible outcomes which might indicate successful consultation or treatment. He may wish for effective cure or treatment of his symptoms; he may want care and concern or reassurance; he may hope to be understood and to be given explanations which he can understand; he may want to find out what he can do to help himself. He may hope for one, all or none of these (and maybe other outcomes too) at different points in the treatment process. The practitioner, on the other hand, may not always be able to, or feel it is appropriate to, satisfy the patient's wants. In any case, she has a duty not to assume that she knows best but rather to remain alert to and respectful of the patient's wishes. Within a relationship of mutual respect, it becomes possible for the patient and practitioner to decide together what is the ultimate objective of treatment, thereby increasing the probability that whatever intervention is made will be relevant and genuinely helpful to the patient.

REFERENCES

Anderson W, O'Connor B B, MacGregor R R, Schwartz J S 1993 Patient use and assessment of conventional and alternative therapies for HIV infection and AIDS. AIDS 7:561–566
Cartwright A 1967 Patients and their doctors. Routledge and Kegan Paul, London
Cartwright A, Anderson R 1981 General practice revisited. Tavistock Publications, London
Cassileth B R, Lusk E J, Strouse T B, Bedenheimer B A 1984 Contemporary unorthodox treatments in cancer medicine. Annals of Internal Medicine 101:105–112
Consumer Advisory Panel, Exeter and District Community Trust 1997 Listen to this. Pavilion Publishing, Brighton
Croft S, Beresford P 1993 Getting involved – a practice manual. Open Services Project and Joseph Rowntree Foundation, London
Coulter A 1994 Assembling the evidence. In: Dunning M, Needham G (eds) But will it work, doctor? Consumer Health Information Consortium, London pp 22–26
Downer S M, Cody M M, McCluskey P et al 1994 Pursuit and practice of complementary therapies by cancer patients receiving conventional treatment. British Medical Journal 309:86–89
Fulder S 1996 The handbook of complementary medicine. Oxford University Press, Oxford
Gilligan C 1982 In a different voice: psychological theory and women's development. Harvard University Press, Boston, Mass

Gilligan C, Ward J V, Taylor, M C 1988 Mapping the moral domain. Harvard University Press, Boston, Mass

Hand R 1989 Alternative therapies used by patients with AIDS. New England Journal of Medicine 320(10): 672–673

Howe D 1993 On being a client. Sage, London

Kai J 1996 Parents' difficulties and information needs in coping with acute illness in preschool children: a qualitative study. British Medical Journal 309:86–89

Langewitz W, Ruttimann S, Laifer G, Maurer P, Kiss A 1994 The integration of alternative treatment modalities in HIV infection – the patient's perspective. Journal of Psychosomatic Research 38(7):687–693

Ley P 1988 Communicating with patients: improving communication, satisfaction and compliance. Croom Helm, London

McIver S 1993 Obtaining the views of users of primary and community health care services. King's Fund Centre, London

Mental Health Foundation 1997 Knowing our own minds. Mental Health Foundation, London

Mitchell A (in press) Complementary therapies in mental health. In: Bailey D (ed) At the core of mental health practice: key issues for practitioners, managers and mental health trainers. Pavilion Press, Brighton

Mooney G 1994 What else do we want from our health services? Social Science and Medicine 39(2):151–154

Murray J, Shepherd S 1993 Alternative or additional medicine? An exploratory study in general practice. Social Science and Medicine 37(8):983–988

Rees-Lewis J C 1994 Patient views on quality care in general practice: literature review. Social Science and Medicine 39(30):655–671

Sharma U 1992 Complementary medicine today: practitioners and patients. Routledge, London

Shifrin K 1995 Squaring the circle: the core syllabus of the British Acupuncture Accreditation Board. Complementary Therapies in Medicine 3:13–15

Sowden A J, Sheldon T A, Alberti G 1995 Shared care in diabetes. British Medical Journal 310:142–143

Steptoe A 1991 The links between stress and illness. Journal of Psychosomatic Research 35(6): 633–644

Stevenson C 1995 All things considered. Nursing Times 91(5):44–45

Tuckett D, Boulton M, Olsen C, Williams A 1985 Meetings between experts: an approach to sharing ideas in medical consultations. Tavistock Publications, London

Vincent C, Furnham A 1996 Why do patients turn to complementary medicine? An empirical study. British Journal of Clinical Psychology 35:37–48

5

Communication and illness: the meaning of illness for patients

COMMUNICATION IN THE CONSULTATION

A consultation with a practitioner is only one step in the process whereby patients attempt to deal with symptoms of illness. People have their own ways of tackling illness: they will attempt self-diagnosis and treatment, they will consult with family members, friends and colleagues and perhaps with pharmacists or non-medical 'experts'. It is only when self, or lay, understanding and treatment are unsuccessful (when symptoms remain unchanged or deteriorate) that the person seeks a consultation with a medical expert (either conventional or non-conventional). Available research in this area has been limited to Western conventional treatment. Calnan (1988) concluded that it is uncertainty which primarily sends people to their GP and satisfaction is 'expressed in terms of the ability of the doctor to listen to the patient's wishes and to communicate information about what was wrong and what treatment was required' (Calnan 1988: 932). However, once the patient reaches the practitioner's consulting room there are frequently difficulties in establishing effective communication. This may, in part, reflect different expectations. It seems that doctors may underestimate patients' desires for explanation and understanding and may emphasize instead the medical treatment itself (Salmon et al 1994). Marsh (1977) found that it was possible to reduce prescriptions for minor illnesses in general practice by giving clearer explanations and recommendations about 'common-sense' self-help activities and noted that when prescriptions were not given, patients were more ready to reveal the real problems that were bothering them.

Ley (1988) found that even when doctors *do* try to keep patients fully informed and to give full and clear explanations, this does not in itself lead to increased patient satisfaction. He concluded that:

It is clear that telling patients is in itself not enough. They have to be told in ways that they can understand and remember, and attempts have to be made to ascertain what the patient's informational needs are. (Ley 1988: 173)

He also found that people are more likely to follow the advice of practitioners when the treatment is understandable and pertinent to them. This finding should alert us to the dangers of uncritically accepting notions of patient–practitioner communication which can be interpreted quite mechanistically unless based on thoughtful analysis of the deeper meanings and purpose of the consultation. Our priority is to encourage practitioners first to clarify *what* communication should be about before dealing with the more technical issue of *how* to talk and listen to patients. Indeed, we believe that a clear framework for the process of treatment should enable practitioners to develop confidence in their own style and ways of being with patients.

Radley (1994) recognized that analysing the consultation as a form of patient–practitioner communication actually falls short of what we are trying to do in attempting to make sense of and enhance what happens in healing relationships. He argued that the concept of 'communication' is at the same time too abstract and too narrowly focused to do justice to the whole range of different things which patients and practitioners wish to achieve within the consultation. The reduction of the consultation to issues of compliance and clarity of explanation, discussed in terms of smoothness and effectiveness, is consistent with a view of the therapeutic relationship which accepts, uncritically, the expert's view of what is, or should be, happening in the consultation. Instead, in this book we are trying to construe the therapeutic relationship as an egalitarian process in which the aims of the consultation and the means by which the aims may be achieved are negotiated between the practitioner and patient. Hence, we take a more patient-centred approach which requires the patient and practitioner to find common ground about problems, needs and priorities in treatment.

SHARED UNDERSTANDING

A major stumbling block in establishing communication is that patients and doctors do not necessarily share the same underlying assumptions: they approach the consultation from different perspectives and have different ways of talking about health and illness.

Different perspectives in the consultation

- Patients often do not know the meanings of the words used by clinicians
- Patients often have their own ideas about illnesses and these often differ from the accepted orthodox ideas
- What the clinician says will be interpreted in terms of the patient's own framework of ideas
- As measured by the patient's own report or by expert judgement, patients often fail to understand what they are told by health care professionals
- Patients are often reluctant to ask for further information even when they would very much like it.

(adapted from Ley 1988: 173)

An important point here is that patients have their own ideas about illness. Other writers (e.g. Kleinman 1988, Stainton Rogers 1991) go much further than Ley and have identified that laypeople have more than ideas: they have their own systematic and coherent theories or models of illness. Such models reflect laypeople's own experiences of health and illness, based on their own everyday lives as well as on information they receive in medical settings, and are set in the context of cultural beliefs about bodies and selves.

Such is the dominance of orthodox medical thinking that it is often assumed that what patients *do* know, whether or not it is biologically accurate, is of no relevance at all (does not even count as knowledge) and so is disregarded in the consultation: it is as if the doctor has a monopoly of expertise. This is the impression of Tuckett et al (1985) who undertook a systematic study of the extent to which ideas are shared in medical consultations. They studied 1303 consultations, conducted by 16 doctors, and interviewed 328 of the patients after consultation. The major findings of relevance were as follows.

Doctors and patients did not manage to achieve a dialogue and so did not share or exchange ideas to a very great degree. Doctors did little to encourage patients to present their views, quite often actively inhibited them from doing so or evaded what patients did say, very rarely explored what a patient was understanding of what they said and did not usually tailor advice and instructions to known details of the patient's life. Moreover, the few attempts made to establish the patient's ideas and explanations were brief to the point of being absent (Tuckett et al 1985: 205).

Overall, they concluded that there was little dialogue, little sharing of ideas and patients were not treated as competent experts in their own health care. In other words, the consultations were carried out on the doctor's terms, not on those of the patient. One result of this was that doctors and patients rarely talked to one another about the consequences of illness or of treatment (such as feelings about the illness, implications for the family or for work). Yet, patients have to manage their lives in terms of coping with these consequences and so are likely to enter a consultation seeking information that will throw light on this.

EXPLANATORY MODELS

The way in which people make sense of illness has been helpfully conceptualized by Kleinman (1988) as 'explanatory models of illness'. The six major themes around which people organize their ideas about the meaning and significance of illness were outlined in Chapter 3. In summary, people consider illness in terms of aetiology, timing, pathology, course of illness, consequences of illness and treatment. The particular ideas any person has about illness are considered to be socially constructed: the ideas are developed through the person's immersion in a culture or society which holds certain beliefs about bodies and selves, and are modified through experiences of health and sickness and through exposure to professional belief systems either as a patient or through training as a practitioner.

Beliefs which underpin or legitimize explanatory models can be used as a framework for making sense of a particular episode of illness and may guide choices about what to do about illness, either as a patient or as a practitioner. It might be expected that, to the extent that both patients and practitioners are grounded in the same culture and thus live in the same world of shared meaning, their conceptual models of illness will also be shared. On the other hand, to the extent that practitioners, through their training and membership of a specialized professional culture, have access to different sets of assumptions, beliefs and knowledge, they will develop 'expert' explanatory models. There is evidence of both overlap and incongruence between biomedical practitioners' and laypersons' explanatory models. In particular, it seems that orthodox medical practitioners and laypeople differ in the extent to which they emphasize somatic or psychosocial aspects of illness: medical practitioners' conceptual models tend to focus around the physical basis of illness, whereas laypeople tend to be relatively more concerned than doctors with the psychological or social aspects of illness.

The different emphases are exemplified in a study by Cohen et al (1994) who interviewed 14 professionals and 39 patients in a diabetes clinic. Although the patients and professionals were similar in many respects (social background, age, level of education) and although the patients had received extensive education from the professionals, there were some important differences between the professionals' and patients' explanatory models. They shared similar views about treatment and severity of illness, but were more discrepant in their views about aetiology and pathophysiology. They emphasized different domains: the professionals saw diabetes as a pathophysiological problem with a primary impact on the patient's body, while patients emphasized difficulties in their social relationships and the impact of diabetes on their everyday lives. Moreover, Cohen's study found that patients had greater access to and awareness of professionals' explanatory models than professionals had of patients' explanatory models. In other words, patients had more understanding of professionals' ways of thinking than professionals had, or used, of laypeople's ways of thinking.

THE IMPACT OF CARTESIAN DUALISM

The prevailing Cartesian dualism of educated Western culture suggests that there is an essential distinction between matter and mind, or between body and soul. Bodies and minds are viewed as separate: in reductive scientific terms, until recently there has been no understood basis in principle for an interaction between the mind and the body. As translated into biomedical practice, there has been a focus on the physical aspects of illness, with diseases being understood as biological phenomena in which signs and symptoms are manifestations of underlying pathology. Social and psychological aspects of illness may have been recognized and viewed as significant in themselves, but there has been no philosophical or theoretical framework for links between the psychosocial and the physical.

Through this conceptual framework it has been possible to treat the body as an object which is separate from the mind. Recent developments in the field of psychoneuroimmunology demonstrate that there are biological mechanisms underpinning links between psychosocial events, such as stressful experiences, and neurological and immunological processes (Steptoe 1991). These findings will take some time to filter into clinical consciousness: in the meantime, Cartesian dualism remains fundamental to positivist biomedicine and impedes treating patients with the recognition that personal meaning and bodily processes are intertwined. Indeed, positive developments within this field await future research. The field of psychoneuroimmunology is still in its infancy and some commentators urge caution. There is evidence that the experience of psychological stress is associated with changes in immune function (Ader 1981). There is further evidence that stress increases susceptibility to infection in the case of the common cold (Cohen et al 1997) and that social support may act as a buffer to vulnerability to infection (Cohen & Wills 1985). However, we must take heed of the warning that, although it seems that severe and chronic stress may well have serious effects on both the immune system and on health, there are few studies which demonstrate clear pathways through events, psychological experience and immune function to illness. The relationships are subtle and complex and there is no justification for uncritical acceptance and unwarranted generalization about the relationship between life events, experience and illness (Evans et al 1997). Nevertheless, psychoneuroimmunology now provides a scientifically respectable conceptual framework within which we can develop a clearer understanding of the relationship between mind and body.

TOUCH, MINDS AND BODIES

Because it pulls together psychological and bodily experiences, touch is experienced as very important in relationships between people in general and within the therapeutic relationship in particular. The use of touch demonstrates and symbolizes our connection with one another, yet can be used in so many ways, both beneficial and harmful: to soothe, calm or comfort, to intervene directly or manipulate, to arouse, stimulate and seduce or to hurt and damage. Vickers (1996) has documented and reviewed some of the evidence and knowledge about touch in treatment, especially in massage and aromatherapy. He noted our limited knowledge about the power and function of touch in treatment and pointed out that the sensitive use of touch often depends on intuition rather than intellect.

It is hard to establish rules which can be applied to such diverse situations as greeting or saying goodbye, engaging in a physical examination, using massage to aid relaxation, comforting a distressed person or helping a dying patient feel at ease. Yet, in each of these situations, touch may be a powerful means of communication, perceived and interpreted differently by each of the participants. The appropriate, sensitive and thoughtful use of touch may enhance verbal communication, building up trust, confidence and rapport, yet, used clumsily, thoughtlessly or invasively, it can inhibit and impair. As always, the practitioner must remain attentive to the patient's own signals when touch is used in treatment.

When patients experience medical care as if their bodies were being dealt with independently of their minds, they complain of being treated impersonally, as unthinking objects. This is in contrast to people's own everyday experience of unity between body and mind or self. We feel ourselves, at least when we are well, to be at one with our bodies: 'it is as if my body *is* myself'. This feeling may break down when we become ill; painful or distorted bodily experience can fragment this inner unity such that the body seems to betray the self, to let us down. It seems that anxiety, at a personal and social level, may heighten this sense of fragmentation between body and self: as we defend ourselves against sometimes intolerable fears about suffering, loss and death we can depersonalize ourselves and others.

Isobel Menzies (1961), in her seminal article 'Social systems as a defence against anxiety', was the first to show how nursing and medical hospital practice tend to be managed in such a way as to protect practitioners from acknowledging the personal aspects of their patients' illnesses. Thornquist (1994) observed in a physiotherapy consultation that the practitioner behaved as if the patient's body was all that was of relevance in the treatment setting, systematically pulling back from talking about personal or social implications or speculations about the illness towards talking of the physical manifestations, consequences and treatment. This was in contrast to the ordinary talk in interviews after the consultation, by patient and practitioner separately, in which there was a sense of taking for granted the integration of body and mind. It seemed that in everyday lay terms, the mind and the body were assumed to be integrated, but in the setting of a physiotherapy consultation, the sense of fragmentation associated with the experience of illness was perpetuated through the concentration of treatment on the body as distinct from the mind.

A scientific framework based on dualism of mind and body and manifested in biomedical treatment cannot provide any sort of framework for patients to ask and explore answers to their personal questions about the significance of their illness for themselves and their lives: 'Why me?', 'Why now?', 'Why this illness?', 'What can I do about it?'.

THE MEANING OF ILLNESS

Good & Good (1982) argued that part of the clinician's task in any therapeutic encounter is to help the patient to make sense of his illness so as to combat demoralization and create new possibilities. This requires the clinician to be able to 'translate' across systems of meaning; in particular, translating between professional and lay models of illness. They argued that healing occurs through this process of negotiation of meaning, but that the importance of understanding has been lost in scientific medicine where symptoms are treated 'as if' they directly, and only, represent somatic states.

Negotiation of meaning requires a broad conceptual framework, which at the very least accepts the possibility of other perspectives. It may be, insofar as holistic models of health and illness transcend mind–body dualism, that they can provide the possibility for patients to develop new understandings of their illnesses within a frame of reference which is relevant for their everyday lives and which takes for granted the interrelatedness of physical, psychological and social events. From what we know of laypeople's explanatory models, practitioners' advice and treatment are more likely to be acceptable and useful to patients if they are framed within understandings which incorporate the psychosocial as well as physical aspects of illness. In practice, this requires practitioners to pay attention to their own and their patients' ideas about what illness and treatment mean in the context of the patient's ordinary life. It may be helpful here to differentiate between three aspects of meaning: meaning as cause; meaning as significance; and meaning as consequence.

Meaning as cause

This is the aspect of meaning in which people try to understand *why* they have become ill or *what has caused their illness*. Cassidy (1995) noted that people differ in the extent to which they view illness as coming from factors outside their awareness and control (e.g. bacteria, viruses, demons, genes) or from factors seen as potentially within the person's awareness and control (general well-being as influenced, for example, by diet, environment and mood). This may be linked with a differentiation between viewing factors causing illness as naturalistic and random (in the sense that no-one could have intended it) or as personalistic and deliberate (in the sense that oneself or someone else could have chosen to make oneself ill).

It has been noted that many complementary health care approaches tend to emphasize the potentially controllable causes of illness within the individual (Oubre 1995). Much is made of the value of encouraging people to take responsibility for maintaining their own health and well-being. There is a danger that too close a focus on ways in which individuals may cause, or be responsible for, their own illness may lead to undesirable consequences. It may redirect attention at a political level away from efforts to understand and ameliorate the social and economic factors associated with ill health. It may also lead, on the one hand, to victim blaming on the part of practitioners who see patients' choices and lifestyles as causing their ill health and, on the other hand, to feelings of guilt and self-blame in patients themselves (Coward 1989). This may be a particular problem for patients with life-threatening disorders such as cancer. People can feel tortured with guilt if they believe, or are led to believe, that aspects of their lives over which they could have had control, such as choices about lifestyle, diet or relationships, were the direct causes of their illness.

One way of tackling this problem of responsibility and causality may be through clarifying the definitions of health and illness and conceptualizing them as separate dimensions instead of viewing them as opposite ends of one dimension (as outlined in Ch. 2). A person *may* have some control over their own health, in the sense of health as development: their capacity to grow, through accommodating to inner and outer events. They are less likely to have control over those events which *happen* to them which may lead to disease, illness and sickness.

The biologist Brian Goodwin pointed out that in the late 20th century the new developments in physics and biology no longer require us to be content with single causes. In complex systems, patterns and organization cannot entirely be predicted from a knowledge of the component parts in isolation:

What is important is to understand the pattern of relationships, of interactions, that exist and how they contribute to the behaviour of the system as an integrated whole. (Goodwin 1994: 168)

Meaning as significance

If we construe health as development, then an important question about illness can become not 'What is its cause?' but 'What is its significance or purpose in terms of the progression of the person's life?'. What message does illness convey to the person about changes they could make in their life? It is important to point out here that for many illnesses, and for many patients, it will not be necessary and, indeed, it will be inappropriate to draw in this sort of question. Some illnesses can indeed be tackled entirely satisfactorily by searching for an isolated cause which can be clearly remedied. This is the case, for example, for those acute or organic disorders for which orthodox medicine can justly claim success. Some patients, too, whatever their illness, will prefer to stay in the realm of what can be known, away from speculation and fantasy. Moreover, as Guggenbühl-Craig & Micklem (1988) argued, some illnesses may be essentially random events: to try to force meaning onto such events through our own desire to control an apparently chaotic universe may violate the patient's own experience of the tragic nature of illness. Sometimes:

The meaning of illness – if it may not be stated in terms of seeming contradiction – is not to search for meaning and turn disaster into good effect, but to withstand and to grapple with the meaninglessness of the tragedy. (Guggenbühl-Craig & Micklem 1988: 150)

However, some patients may very much want to find meaning in their tragedy and will be relieved to have the opportunity to share with the practitioner their feelings and ideas about what the illness could be telling them about changes and developments they might make in their lives. Through questioning the significance of the illness, in an act of creative imagination, the person may develop new insights, further knowledge or greater awareness of themselves which may lead to a change in direction. Thus, the experience of illness could be seen as part of a developmental process through which the person moves towards health, as suggested in Harrison's (1984) popular book *Love your disease, it's keeping you healthy*. Paradoxically, as Tatham (1988) suggested, being ill may be 'healthy' when the illness signifies constructive changes that the person could make in his life.

While this sort of imaginative and creative speculation may be helpful for some patients who come for complementary health care, the opportunity to reflect in this way should only be offered very carefully. It can be seen most constructively as a way of looking forward to what might be done differently in the future, providing a context within which the practitioner could offer relevant treatment and self-help ideas rather than as a way of allowing the patient to berate himself for what he may feel he has done wrong in the past. Moreover, it is essential that the practitioner does not impose onto the patient her views of what the illness could mean. In treatment, if the patient and practitioner come to a shared understanding about the significance of the illness, then the practitioner can use the patient's perspective as a framework for her intervention in order to enable treatment to make more sense for the patient.

Meaning as a consequence

Illnesses obviously vary in their impact on the person's life. Some are transitory with only temporary consequences; others may be chronic, with consequences which never entirely disappear. For patients, the consequences of the illness (and of the treatment) are at the foreground of their awareness. Most people, when asked the question 'What does your illness mean?', will answer immediately in terms of consequences: 'It means I can't go to work', 'I can't dress myself', I can't look after my children in the way that I want to', 'I suffer pain', 'I may die'. Kleinman, in his book *The illness narratives* (1988), emphasized how important it is that practitioners should pay serious attention to the patient's experiences, especially for those who are chronically ill, whose lives are inextricably intertwined with their illness. There are two (at least) important reasons for this.

First, listening seriously to the patient's account of their illness, their suffering, its impact on their lives and on those close to them is in itself part of the therapeutic endeavour.

Legitimating the patient's illness experience – authorizing that experience, auditing it empathically – is a key task in the care of the chronically ill, but one that is particularly difficult to do with the regularity and consistency and sheer perseverance that chronicity necessitates. (Kleinman 1988: 17)

Witnessing, and helping to order, the person's experience of suffering can in itself bring relief. Another orthodox medical practitioner put it in this way: 'Healers can hear pain, healers give people permission to show pain, healers are not afraid to see pain' (Emmanuel 1995: 798).

Second, Kleinman identified that chronic illnesses tend to oscillate between periods of exacerbation or amplification, when symptoms worsen, and periods of quiescence or damping, when the symptoms reduce. He noted that psychological factors (such as anxiety, depression) and social factors (such as poor social support, life changes, impaired personal relationships) are associated with exacerbation of symptoms. On the other hand, the swing towards damping (which he calls 'a kind of internal health-promoting system' and which relates to the complementary practitioner's notion of self-healing) can be associated with strengthened social support, enhanced self-efficacy and rekindled morale.

Attention to the consequences of illness, and their relationship with exacerbation or reduction of symptoms, can direct both patient and practitioner towards practical ways of dealing with these consequences in order to cope more effectively with the illness. Using this approach to treatment, especially with chronic conditions, presents a way of managing illness rather than perpetuating an unrealistic myth of cure. As Kleinman pointed out, in chronic illness the quest for cure is a dangerous myth which distracts attention from the step-by-step behaviours that lessen suffering, even if they do not magically heal the disease. Complementary practitioners may value paying detailed attention to the consequences of illness as a way of focusing on reduction of suffering and promotion of self-care as the primary goal of treatment.

THE PRACTICALITIES OF COMMUNICATION: HOW TO PROMOTE DIALOGUE

The ways in which doctors can assert control through verbal and non-verbal communication have been well documented. Ong et al (1995), in a review of studies of doctor–patient communication, found evidence that the style of relationship in which the doctor has high control, involving asking many questions and interrupting frequently, does not allow the patient to speak at any length. The authors concluded that:

Difference in control in medical communication may stem from the patient's limited understanding of medical problems and treatment, heightened uncertainty, doctors' control of medical information, and the institutionalized roles prescribed for the doctor and patient. (Ong et al 1995: 910)

These issues are important not only for how patients feel or their satisfaction with treatment, but also for actual treatment outcome. Kaplan et al (1989) found that patients with chronic illnesses did better (as measured physiologically, behaviourally or subjectively by the patient's own perception) when there was more patient- and less physician-controlled behaviour, when more emotion (especially negative emotion) was expressed by patient and physician and when more information was given by the physician in response to information seeking by the patient.

It is striking that it is the question of control of information which seems extremely important for patients. Patients are frequently dissatisfied with the information they receive; in one finding, doctors underestimated patients' desires for information in 65% of encounters (Waitzkin 1984). It is less clear whether patients wish to take a more active part in decision making about their treatment. The findings here are discrepant: for example, most patients with a long-standing illness such as cancer have been reported to want decisions about their treatment to be made by the doctor, yet the converse was true for patients with newly diagnosed cancer (Buetow 1995).

Nichols (1993) gives some vivid examples of the ways in which patients can be confused and frightened by insufficient or conflicting communication and how they can be made to feel foolish or naughty when they attempt to clarify the information. Sometimes the problems of communication occur when there are several health care staff dealing with the patient and it is more difficult to get a consistent set of information together.

For the complementary practitioner, the situation with the patient may be more like the consultation between GP, or consultant, and patient, which has been described in Pendleton et al's (1984) book *The consultation: an approach to learning and teaching*. Here, the authors describe stages in the process of the consultation which centre around the patient's involvement in the interaction. The tasks in the consultation are as follows.

1. To define the reason for the patient's attendance, including the nature and history of the problems, their aetiology, the patient's ideas, concerns and expectations, and the effects of the problems.
2. To consider other problems such as continuing problems and risk factors.
3. To choose, with the patient, an appropriate action for each problem.
4. To achieve a shared understanding of the problems with the patient.
5. To involve the patient in the management and encourage him to accept appropriate responsibility.
6. To use time and resources appropriately in the consultation and in the long term.
7. To establish and maintain a relationship with the patient within which to achieve the other tasks.

(from Pendleton et al 1984: 41–49)

The interaction between patient and practitioner can be examined from the viewpoint of social psychology and non-verbal communication. Michael Argyle's book *Bodily communication* (1988) covers almost every aspect of how we infer feelings from gestures, expressions, movements and vocal behaviour. In successful interactions there is synchrony of speech, acknowledgement of bodily space, dissociation of highly emotive topics of speech from other emotive communication such as touch, bodily exposure or protracted eye contact, an appropriate power balance through seating at the same height, similar volumes of speech and gestures to involve the other person in the flow of the encounter. The physical environment can have a large impact on the comfort of the patient and the creation of a conducive environment for easy interaction: spacing of furniture, colour of decor, level of lighting and soundproofing can be extremely important in influencing people's desires to engage in honest and open communication.

IMPLICATIONS FOR PRACTICE

1. Good communication takes place in the context of a respectful and caring therapeutic relationship. The tasks of the practitioner are:

- to negotiate an authentic relationship which may change over time and which is suited to the needs of the particular individual
- to listen carefully to what the patient wants to communicate (both with words and with his body)
- to offer support, encouragement and realistic hope
- to be sensitive to the patient's emotional state and needs.

2. Good communication between patient and practitioner requires the ability to take the other person's perspective into account. The practitioner should try to find out the patient's explanatory model of illness by asking for his beliefs, thoughts and feelings. Patients' answers to questions are unlikely to be consistent or clear: there will be different layers of ideas and beliefs which may be more or less accessible, or buried in the fears and anxieties associated with illness. The challenge in the consultation is to clarify the patient's views about:

- what might have caused the illness
- what was significant when the symptoms began
- what the illness is
- what the future might hold
- what treatment might be needed.

3. The practitioner should also try to convey to the patient her explanatory model, at a pace and level which is relevant to the patient's understanding and desire to know. It is best to do this using the patient's language, wherever possible, using words and metaphors which will be accessible to him. The practitioner should explain her views about:

- the cause of the illness (if cause is relevant and can be identified; if not, explain why not)
- the treatment which is recommended
- what self-help activities the patient can undertake
- what might be the consequences of treatment (expected outcome, possible side-effects, limitations and timescale).

4. Good communication includes trying to understand the person's experiences of the consequences of his illness. Serious attention should be given to the patient's account of the history of his illness.

- What are the important events and relationships in his life?
- What consequences does the illness have for his life (everyday activities, family life, social relationships, work)?
- What consequences might treatment have for his life?
- May any unwanted consequences discourage the patient from using treatment and self-help activities?

5. Clear, open and respectful communication provides a framework for a shared understanding between patient and practitioner, which will change and develop over time. This may enable the patient to:

- decide whether the treatment offered is relevant for his needs
- make use of treatment and self-help recommendations because they have been explained in a way which is relevant to his understanding
- feel helped by the practitioner's support, understanding and acceptance.

REFERENCES

Ader R 1981 Psychoneuroimmunology. Academic Press, New York
Argyle M 1988 Bodily communication, 2nd edn. Routledge, London
Buetow S A 1995 What do general practitioners and the patients want from general practice and are they receiving it? A framework. Social Science and Medicine 40:213–221

Calnan M 1988 Towards a conceptual framework of lay evaluation of health care. Social Science and Medicine 27:927–933

Cassidy C M 1995 Social science theory and methods in the study of alternative and complementary medicine. Journal of Alternative and Complementary Medicine 1(1):19–40

Cohen S, Wills T A 1985 Stress, social support and the buffering hypothesis. Psychological Bulletin 98:310–357

Cohen M Z, Tripp-Reimer T, Smith C, Sorofman B, Lively S 1994 Explanatory models of diabetes: patient-practitioner variation. Social Science and Medicine 38(1):59–66

Cohen S, Doyle W J, Skoner D P, Rabin B S, Gwaltrey J M 1997 Social ties and susceptibility to the common cold. Journal of the American Medical Association 277(24):1940–1944

Coward R 1989 The whole truth: the myth of alternative health. Faber and Faber, London

Emmanuel L 1995 The privilege and the pain. Annals of Internal Medicine 122:797 798

Evans P, Clow A, Hucklebridge F 1997 Stress and the immune system. The Psychologist 10(7):303–307

Good B J, Good M D 1982 The meaning of symptoms: a cultural hermeneutic model for clinical practice. In: Eisenberg L, Kleinman A (eds) The relevance of social science for medicine. Reidel, Dordrecht

Goodwin B 1994 How the leopard changed its spots. Weidenfeld and Nicolson, London

Guggenbühl-Craig A, Micklem N 1988 No answer to Job: reflections on the limitations of meaning in illness. In: Kidel M, Rowe-Leetes S (eds) The meaning of illness. Routledge, London

Harrison J W 1984 Love your disease, it's keeping you healthy. Angus and Robertson, London

Kaplan S H, Greenfields S, Ware J E 1989 Assessing the effects of physician–patient interactions on the outcomes of chronic disease. Medical Care 27(3):S110–S127

Kleinman A 1988 The illness narratives. Basic Books, New York

Ley P 1988 Communicating with patients: improving communication, satisfaction and compliance. Croom Helm, London

Marsh G N 1977 'Curing' minor illness in general practice. British Medical Journal 2:1267–1269

Menzies E P 1961 The functioning of social systems as a defence against anxiety. Tavistock Pamphlet No 3. Tavistock Publications, London

Nichols K A 1993 Psychological care in physical illness, 2nd edn. Chapman and Hall, London

Ong L M L, DeHaes J C J M, Hoos A M, Lammes F B 1995 Doctor–patient communication: a review of the literature. Social Science and Medicine 40:903–918

Oubre A 1995 Social context of complementary medicine in Western society. Journal of Alternative and Complementary Medicine 1(1):41–56

Pendleton D, Schofield T, Tate P, Havelock P 1984 The consultation: an approach to learning and teaching. Oxford University Press, Oxford

Radley A 1994 Making sense of illness: the social psychology of health and disease. Sage, London

Salmon P, Sharma N, Valori R, Bellenger N 1994 Patients' intentions in primary care: relationships to physical and psychological symptoms, and their perception by general practitioners. Social Science and Medicine 38(4):585–592

Stainton Rogers W 1991 Explaining health and illness. Harvester Wheatsheaf, Hemel Hempstead

Steptoe A 1991 The links between stress and illness. Journal of Psychosomatic Research 35(6):633–644

Tatham P 1988 Items and motion. In: Kidel M, Rowe-Leetes S (eds) The meaning of illness, Routledge, London

Thornquist E 1994 Profession and life: separate worlds. Social Science and Medicine 39(5):701–713

Tuckett D, Boulton M, Olsen C, Williams A 1985 Meetings between experts: an approach to sharing ideas in medical consultations. Tavistock Publications, London

Vickers A 1996 Massage and aromatherapy: a guide for health professionals. Chapman and Hall, London

Waitzkin H 1984 Doctor–patient communication. Clinical implications of social scientific research. Journal of the American Medical Association 252:2441–2446

6

What makes change happen in treatment?

Practitioners of all traditions tend to assume that it is the techniques they use which lead to change for patients. Indeed, practitioners make so much investment, in terms of time, money and effort in acquiring the knowledge and skills of their chosen discipline, that it would be surprising if they were not highly committed to a belief in the effectiveness of their techniques. So much so that, when it is found that a large proportion of change for patients cannot be explained by the use of techniques alone, such effects tend to be dismissed into a dustbin category and labelled placebo effects or spontaneous recovery, as if they were somehow less significant or less valuable than change which could be attributed to technical intervention alone. However, change is no less real because it comes through unexpected, unintended or unexplained means. Indeed, it is possible to turn the argument on its head and propose that in most treatments, irrespective of theoretical framework or techniques used, it is the non-technical factors which are central to healing.

WHAT IS THE EVIDENCE OF THE EFFECTIVENESS OF NON-TECHNICAL FACTORS IN HEALING?

There are three lines of evidence which support the proposition that factors beyond the specific treatment techniques account for a significant proportion of change for patients. First are the placebo studies in medical (biomedical) treatments, second are psychotherapy outcome studies and third are observations of 'spontaneous remission'.

Placebo effects in medical treatments

The derivation of the word 'placebo' from the Latin 'I shall be pleasing' and its definition in the *Oxford English Dictionary* as 'a flatterer, sycophant, parasite', as well as 'an epithet given to any medicine adapted more to please than to benefit the patient', serve to convey the impression that the use of placebo implies disreputable trickery on the part of the practitioner. However, studies of medical treatment demonstrate that, in fact, the placebo is ubiquitous: it operates whether or not the practitioner intends its use and thus there is more to any treatment than seems apparent on the surface.

A thorough and sophisticated definition of placebo, provided by Shapiro, is:

... any therapeutic procedure (or that component of any therapeutic procedure) which is given deliberately to have an effect, or unknowingly has an effect on a patient, symptoms, syndrome or disease, but which is objectively without specific activity for the condition being treated. The therapeutic procedure may be given with or without conscious knowledge that the procedure is a placebo, may be an active (non-inert) or non-active (inert) procedure, and includes therefore all medical procedures no matter how specific – oral and parenteral medication, topical preparations, inhalants, and mechanical, surgical, and psychological procedures. The placebo must be differentiated from the placebo effect which may or may not occur and which may be favourable or unfavourable. The placebo effect is defined as the changes produced by placebos. (Shapiro 1960)

Watts (1992) makes the point that it is neither the specific treatment nor the placebo which facilitates change. The placebo effect is always present, whether or not the specific treatment itself is beneficial.

At first sight, the evidence is quite startling: it is well documented now that actual, observable, measurable, physical changes can be obtained when doctors and/or patients believe an active medication or intervention has been given when actually the intervention was technically inert. Placebo intervention, whether administered knowingly or inadvertently, may have an effect on practically any organ system in the body (Benson & Epstein 1975). Placebo benefits have been reported in a whole range of conditions including post-operative pain, angina pectoris, cough, headache, peptic ulcer, essential hypertension, seasickness, anxiety, tension and degenerative arthritis (Helman 1990, Turner et al 1994).

One of the most dramatic descriptions of the placebo effect in practice was in a study conducted earlier this century and reported by Benson & McCallie (1979). In a double-blind clinical trial to evaluate a surgical procedure, patients with angina pectoris received 'mock surgery' (an anaesthetic and skin incision but no technical surgical intervention) or 'real' surgery (ligation of the internal mammary artery). On almost all measures, patients who believed that they had been given the surgical intervention did as well or even better than those who actually did receive the intervention.

Subsequently, numerous investigations have confirmed that symptoms can change, sometimes dramatically, even when a supposed active agent turns out not to be actually present. Another example was a study by Hashish et al (1988) which looked at outcomes of ultrasound treatment (an established effective treatment) following wisdom tooth extraction when, unknown to the therapist, the ultrasound machine was turned on or off. The placebo condition turned out to be highly effective in decreasing pain and reducing swelling: in other words, patients' symptoms improved whether or not they actually received the ultrasound treatment which they and the therapists thought that they were getting. Placebos can alter symptoms negatively as well as positively. They can create toxic side-effects (the so-called nocebo effect): a range of placebo side-effects were documented by Beecher (1955), including nausea, headache and drowsiness. At a more dramatic level, voodoo death demonstrates the powerful nature of expectation of harm.

We can be left in no doubt that physiological and psychological change, both beneficial and deleterious, can and does follow interventions which are technically inert. Indeed, the enormous intellectual and scientific effort put into controlling for placebo effects in drug trials bears witness to the practical reality of the phenomenon. From a purely rational cause and effect perspective, the placebo effect seems remarkable, curious and puzzling – how is it that change can happen when the agent which is supposed to cause the change is not actually present? Clearly, something complicated must be going on. And indeed, research indicates that this is so: investigations of the mode of action of placebos demonstrate that their effectiveness lies, at least in part, in the nature of the interaction between patient and practitioner. It is often said that up to one-third of patients improve under placebo conditions; this figure was based on observations by Beecher (1955) but more recent reviews (Wall 1992) indicate that responders to placebos range from none to all patients, depending on the conditions of the trial.

The placebo effect is most powerful under the following conditions:

- when the patient expects it to work
- when the practitioner expects it to work
- when it is administered by someone viewed as high status by the patient
- when it appears to be a credible treatment
- when it is presented as a major or ostensibly powerful treatment.

(Richardson 1989)

In her thorough analysis of the role of placebo factors in pain management, Skevington concluded that:

Quintessentially, [the placebo effect] is a sociopsychological phenomenon, because it integrates the patient's beliefs and expectations about the treatment received with those of the person who administered the treatment and the situation or context in which this exchange took place. (Skevington 1995: 261)

At first sight, acknowledgement of the placebo effect can lead to therapeutic nihilism: if change occurs irrespective of technical intervention, practitioners may ask, 'Why bother with technique at all?'. However, just because change can and does happen in the absence of technical intervention, this does not imply that the placebo effect can account for *all* change. It may well be that the non-specific effects of treatment cannot operate in the absence of a credible (to both patient and practitioner) technique. We need a sophisticated understanding of the complexity of the treatment act, elaborated in Chapter 3. No *one* component of treatment can exist in isolation: the task of the practitioner is to pull together techniques with theory and practical action into a whole, made coherent and significant within the therapeutic relationship.

Psychotherapy outcome studies

There are many approaches to helping people with emotional and psychological difficulties. At first sight, the approaches differ dramatically in both their rationales and their treatment methods. Techniques used include sharing feelings with an empathic and reflective listener (as in person-centred counselling), more active, cathartic expressions of emotion (such as in Gestalt therapy) or interpretation to connect current experiences with formative experiences in childhood (used in psychodynamic therapy). In more prescriptive therapies (such as behaviour therapy or cognitive therapy), people are facilitated more directly to change their behaviours or their thoughts and beliefs, through specific strategies and tasks. Treatment may take place individually or within group settings. Psychological therapies may be carried out effectively by highly trained, long-experienced professionals or by volunteers or lay helpers.

The research evidence indicates that most therapies used are more effective than no treatment, whether conducted by highly trained or lay people (Barkham 1996, Elton Wilson & Barkham 1994). One review suggested that, typically, psychotherapy clients will fare better than 75% of untreated people (Smith & Glass 1977). However, despite the clear differences between approaches, psychotherapies all produce comparable outcomes: most outcome research reviews show little or no differential effectiveness of different psychotherapies (Stiles et al 1986). This presents a paradox: why should such apparently different approaches have broadly similar results? One possibility is that the research studies are insufficiently detailed. It may be that, in any study of one particular therapy, grouping together different practitioners and different patients, each with their own particular problems, produces broad generalized outcome findings which simply mask the individual differences. Moreover, different treatments may be expected to lead to different outcomes, especially when we consider that psychological well-being varies enormously; indeed, effective therapy may lead to greater differentiation between people in terms of spontaneity, creativity, control, choice and self-actualization. Thus, outcome measures simply considering 'global improvement' may be too general and may miss specific changes more highly valued by the patients themselves.

The questions to be asked should be more detailed, as suggested by Paul (1967): not simply 'Is treatment effective?' but 'What treatment, by whom, is most effective for this individual with that specific problem and under which circumstances?' (Paul 1967: 111), to which we may add 'Leading to what outcomes?'. Stiles et al (1986) noted that while Paul's approach appeared promising, the results over 20 years are sparse. Despite a few specific findings that particular therapies are more helpful for particular problems (such as behaviour therapy for obsessional disorders), by and large the conclusion remains the same: the outcomes of different psychotherapies with clinical populations are equivalent.

Perhaps, then, the therapy techniques are not as different as they claim to be: perhaps therapists from different orientations actually do quite similar things in treatment. Stiles (1979) explored whether therapists practised techniques appropriate to their theoretical approach. He found that 80–90% of the things which therapists said to patients conformed to their particular theoretical positions. For example, client-centred therapists used non-directive modes (reflection and acknowledgement) while Gestalt therapists used directive modes (advice, question, disclosure). The paradox remains: therapists do employ different techniques, yet the beneficial end result remains the same.

The conclusion which most investigators have reached is that there must be some common features shared by all psychotherapies which underlie or override differences in techniques and that it is these common features, or non-specific factors, rather than the techniques alone, which are responsible for beneficial change.

What are the non-specific factors in psychotherapy?

It seems that it is what the patient and practitioner each bring in their commitment to therapy and expectation of effectiveness, and the relationship which develops between them which provides the core ingredients for therapeutic change. For the patient, Stiles et al (1986) concluded that patients do best if they have moderate expectations for success, whereas unrealistically high or low expectations are associated with poorer outcomes. They also found that patients who benefit most from therapy are those who become most actively involved in making positive contributions during treatment.

The best known statement of what the therapist should provide is the triad of 'necessary and sufficient conditions for change' formulated by Rogers (1957):

- warmth (unconditional positive regard)
- empathy (accurate understanding)
- genuineness (openness).

In practice, it seems that these qualities cannot be independently rated but rather that they depend on the patient's perception of the therapist within the therapeutic relationship, where the qualities merge together into an overall impression of a 'good therapist' (Sloane et al 1975).

What seems most important of all for change is the relationship between the therapist and the patient or the 'therapeutic alliance'. From this perspective, techniques, theories and tasks are relatively unimportant except as vehicles for the therapeutic relationship. Here again, we must remind ourselves of the holistic nature of the treatment act: treatment which did away with technique, theory and action and relied solely on the therapeutic relationship would be as ephemeral as the smile on Alice in Wonderland's disappearing cat! The therapeutic relationship must be offered within a purposeful context or it would be divested of its meaning.

Strupp (1989), in his review of what the research evidence can teach the psychotherapy practitioner, concluded that change in treatment is through a 'corrective emotional experience' in the therapeutic relationship. His formulation was as follows. First, the practitioner provides an empathic context in which the patient is accepted and listened to respectfully. Then she tries to understand and deal (in a non-entangled, flexible and adaptive way) with the patient's 'enactments' in therapy. That is, she notices, but does not react to, the emotional response in herself which is evoked when the patient behaves towards her in particular ways which may actually derive from the patient's own past experiences. Instead, she tries to *respond*, rather than *react to* the patient's needs, in such a way that the patient's self-esteem is kept intact or enhanced, while the patient is freed to develop new patterns of interaction.

Transference and countertransference

In his account of the nature of the change in the therapeutic process, Strupp (1989) has drawn on the notions of transference and countertransference which are central concepts in psychoanalytic treatment. At its simplest, transference is the ordinary human tendency to transfer feelings and action patterns from one significant personal relationship to another. Countertransference is the set of complementary feelings and actions which are 'pulled out' in response to another person's transference. It has been thought, within the psychoanalytic tradition, that the powerful experiences of early infancy and childhood may tend particularly to be replayed and perpetuated in those later relationships characterized by dependency on the one side and authority on the other.

Insofar as these ways of feeling and behaving (and other people's response to them) may contribute to the maintenance of patterns of being which relate to the person's illness or distress, then it is important that therapists and practitioners try not to be drawn into reacting automatically in accordance with the patient's usual expectations. It is useful for the practitioner to note what the patient's transference may draw out of her (countertransference), while yet respectfully and thoughtfully retaining her own clarity and perspective.

The crucial importance of the relationship in psychotherapy

The view of the therapeutic relationship as the central factor in psychotherapy accords with the views of patients themselves. Sloane et al (1975) carried out a study in which the outcomes of treatment given by psychodynamically oriented therapists were compared to outcomes for behaviourally orientated therapists. Although there were some clear and measurable differences in outcome between the therapies, both were extremely successful: the main presenting symptom improved for about 90% of the patients. When asked what they had found to be helpful in their treatment, most patients, regardless of their treatment approach, rated these statements as very important:

- the personality of your doctor
- her helping you to understand your problems
- encouraging you gradually to practise facing the things that bother you
- being able to talk to an understanding person
- helping you to understand yourself.

Thus, for patients in treatment, relationship, understanding, encouragement and responsibility emerge as the key issues.

Influential writers on psychotherapy have emphasized the essentially personal nature of the therapeutic enterprise. Smail (1978), in his book *Psychotherapy: a personal approach*, saw therapy as a process beginning with clarification and negotiation of meaning, so that patient and therapist can reach a shared under-standing of the nature of the patient's problems, and proceeding through the experience, within the therapeutic relationship, of risk, terror, agony and despair before change can be made. He suggested that psychotherapy can do no more than help free somebody to pursue his existence or, in other words, to facilitate his continued development. Peter Lomas (1981), another dis-tinguished psychotherapist, described healing in a similar way, as 'promoting growth in others'.

Spontaneous remission

There is a well-recognized phenomenon of spontaneous remission, in a range of illnesses, in which patients recover without any apparent intervention. This is exemplified in people with addictions. Orford (1985) made a thorough investigation of the processes that may lead to change in those who have excessive appetites or addictions, whether to alcohol, food, drugs or sex. In terms of the particular treatments for excessive appetites, there is a comparable story to that of medical treatments overall and psychotherapy in particular: each new treatment has its own rationale and is pursued vigorously, optimistically and apparently effectively but turns out, when used routinely, to have a similar, moderate, level of success as did previous therapies. Success rates average about one-third (in a range of 20–45%) after 6–12 months following treatment and different treatments tend to produce very similar results.

Orford went on to look further at those people who give up their addictions without formal help and found that, indeed, substantial numbers of people do well in the absence of any specialist therapy. Such change is often called 'spontaneous remission': a misnomer, in Orford's view, since it implies that what goes on in treatment is what really counts and what occurs elsewhere is somehow less substantial or important. Finding out what happens when people are able to give up their addictions on their own may cast light on what happens in formal treat-ment. Treatment could be viewed as a way of strengthening or formalizing those beneficial processes which may be available to some people in their everyday lives, providing another perspective on the idea of non-technical processes in treatment.

The change process is essentially social: it seems that people first make a personal commitment to change which is activated by some important social event (maybe recognition of hurt to others or an acceptance of advice from someone at a critical moment of readiness), which is then turned into sustained resolution and maintenance of change through interactions with others. Orford quoted at length Bacon's conclusions about the everyday social nature of the recovery process (in this case, recovery from drinking) as follows:

The recovery personnel of prime significance are the associates, the significant others. Perhaps medical or welfare or religious or law enforcement personnel are essential at this stage, are necessary requirements for the treatment process even to begin, but the crucial persons for recovery are the daily life associates through time, not the specialists during 'formal' treatment periods.

The treatment methods crucial for recovery ... are those processes and structures and interrelationships and attitudes and behaviours of the person and of the relevant surrounding others which rebuild control ... recovery itself comprises the moulding of such changes into a pattern of life, life through time, life with meaningful others, life more satisfying to the person, to his associates, and to the community. It is that moulding through time, persons, and society which is the core of the treatment. (Bacon 1973)

Orford himself put treatment firmly into context:

It is the individual's day-to-day world and the decisions he or she takes to accommodate to it or to change it that are primary, and it is within that framework that expert treatment plays its modest part. (Orford 1985: 269).

These observations on the possibility of change in ordinary life give support to Lomas' (1981) view of therapy as a particular form of friendship: a way of facilitating change, growth or development when extra resources are needed.

COMPONENTS OF THE CHANGE PROCESS: IMPLICATIONS FOR PRACTICE

The most important lesson to be drawn from this chapter is that change is essentially a social process, which may or may not take place in a formal treatment setting. It is possible to draw out three aspects of the change process which require attention:

1. commitment by the person undergoing change
2. facilitation through some sort of external leverage
3. maintenance through social interaction.

Let us consider the implications of each of these when a person consults a practitioner for help. Change in this account implies change in the broadest sense as outlined in the model of treatment in Chapter 3: it may mean change in symptoms or behaviour, in beliefs, in feelings or in the capacity to look after oneself.

Commitment by the patient

Commitment involves a decision to look for help, a commitment to treatment and the treatment ritual.

The decision to look for help

This takes place before the patient reaches the consulting room; turning to a practitioner may be only one step in a sequence of attempts at self-help, following involvement of family, friends and others in considering possibilities for action. There may be some trial and error in finding help and any individual patient may find help from a variety of sources.

Contributing to the treatment process

This may be personal, such as telling his story, describing his symptoms or submitting to a physical examination, or may be financial or practical, in terms of paying fees, giving up time and making the effort to reach the practitioner's consulting room.

Participating in ritual

Ritual symbolizes the involvement of the patient in treatment and structures the meaning of the encounter (Helman 1990). In healing rituals, the attention to the importance of the occasion, its difference from ordinary life and the power of the practitioner (symbolized by the various signs of her status, such as careful apportioning of time, her clothing, certificates on the wall, her specialized tools, particular use of language and her ritualized behaviour) all convey to the patient, and indeed to the practitioner, a sense that change can be made to happen through the activities inherent within the ritual. Participation in the ritual may itself draw the patient into participation in the healing process.

Moreover, rituals may signal to the wider social world that the patient has entered a process of change; they may act as a way of engaging the patient's later participation in the maintenance of change.

Facilitation of change

Change which takes place in the treatment setting may involve all or any of the following: feelings, beliefs, behaviours and symptoms.

Change in feelings

The practitioner's offer of hope, encouragement and reassurance may enhance the patient's morale. The experience of a therapeutic relationship with someone who offers care and concern may raise the patient's self-esteem, while the process of telling the story may release for the patient the expression of pent-up emotions.

Change in beliefs

The practitioner's demonstration or conviction that there are things which the patient can do to help himself may act to change the patient's own sense of self-efficacy: that is, his belief in his personal effectiveness. Moreover, the conceptual framework offered by the practitioner may help the patient to see his problems in a new light and generate new possibilities for action.

Change in behaviours

Within the treatment encounter, the patient may be encouraged to try out new ways of behaving, either interpersonally, such as developing new social skills, new ways of communicating or new ways of expressing feelings, or individually, such as through new movement or posture patterns.

Change in symptoms

The techniques applied by the practitioner may act directly to relieve or alter the patient's physical symptoms.

Maintenance of change

Any changes which are made within the treatment setting can only be beneficial and lasting if they can be maintained and generalized into the patient's everyday world. There are two implications of importance here.

Personal responsibility

Wills (1982) argued that part of the therapeutic task is to attribute change to the patient's own actions, conveying that it is the patient who has solved the problem, not the practitioner.

Support from others

Those people who are important in the patient's everyday life are in a position to help to maintain (or, indeed, sabotage) any changes which he may make. Permanent recovery (whether this means 'cure' or satisfactory coping with chronic illness) requires moulding changes into ordinary life. Whenever possible, the therapist should help the patient to identify ways in which his world and the people in it can adapt to help him maintain the changes he makes, while at the same time acknowledging that some aspects of the person's life cannot be altered. Thus, change efforts can be realistic.

SUMMARY

In most treatments, factors other than the specific techniques of the approach are central to healing. Evidence for this comes from the placebo effect, from studies of outcome in psychotherapy and from instances of spontaneous remission of symptoms. The non-specific factors in treatment are essentially within the practitioner–patient relationship and involve a genuine inter-action, an acceptance of the patient by the practitioner and an ability to understand the problem from the patient's point of view. There are broad-ranging implications for practice and scope for development of the effectiveness of treatments through attention to the therapeutic relationship.

REFERENCES

Bacon S 1973 The process of addiction to alcohol: social aspects. Quarterly Journal of Studies on Alcohol 34:1–27

Barkham M 1996 Individual psychotherapy: process and outcome findings across successive research generations. In: Dryden W (ed) Handbook of individual therapy, 3rd edn. Sage, London, pp 328–364

Beecher H K 1955 The powerful placebo. Journal of the American Medical Association 159:1602–1606

Benson H, Epstein M D 1975 The placebo effect: a neglected asset in the care of patients. Journal of the American Medical Association 232:1225–1227

Benson H, McCallie D P 1979 Angina pectoris and the placebo effect. New England Journal of Medicine 300:1424–1428

Elton Wilson J, Barkham M 1994 A practitioner-scientist approach to psychotherapy process and outcome research. In: Clarkson P, Pokorny M R (eds) Handbook of psychotherapy. Routledge, London, pp 49–72

Hashish I, Feinman C, Harvey W 1988 Reduction of postoperative pain and swelling by ultra sound: a placebo effect. Pain 83:303–311

Helman C G 1990 Culture, health and illness, 2nd edn. Butterworth Heinemann, Oxford

Lomas P 1981 The case for a personal psychotherapy. Oxford University Press, Oxford

Orford J 1985 Excessive appetites: a psychological view of addictions. Wiley, Chichester

Paul G L 1967 Strategy of outcome research in psychotherapy. Journal of Consulting Psychology 31:109–118

Richardson P 1989 Placebos: their effectiveness and modes of action. In: Broome A K (ed) Health psychology: processes and applications. Chapman and Hall, London

Rogers C R 1957 The necessary and sufficient conditions of therapeutic personality change. Journal of Consulting Psychology 21:95–103

Shapiro A K 1960 A contribution to a history of the placebo effect. Behavioral Science 5:109–135

Skevington S M 1995 Psychology of pain. Wiley, Chichester

Sloane R B, Staples F R, Cristol A H, Yorkston, N J, Whipple K 1975 Psychotherapy versus behaviour therapy. Harvard University Press, Cambridge, Mass

Smail D J 1978 Psychotherapy: a personal approach. Dent, London

Smith M L, Glass G V 1977 Meta-analysis of psychotherapy outcome studies. American Psychologist 32:752–760

Stiles W B 1979 Verbal response modes and psychotherapeutic technique. Psychiatry 42:49–62

Stiles W B, Shapiro D A, Elliott R 1986 Are all psychotherapies equivalent? American Psychologist 41:165–180

Strupp H H 1989 Psychotherapy: can the practitioner learn from the researcher? American Psychologist 44:717–724

Turner J A, Richard A D, Loeser J D, von Korff M, Fordyce W E 1994 The importance of placebo effects in pain treatment and research. Journal of the American Medical Association 271(20):1609–1614

Wall P D 1992 The placebo effect: an unpopular topic. Pain 51:1–3

Watts G 1992 Pleasing the patient. Faber and Faber, London

Wills T A 1982 Nonspecific factors in helping relationships. In: Wills T A (ed) Basic processes in helping relationships. Academic Press, New York, ch 17, p 381

7

Power in treatment

DISCOMFORT AND AMBIVALENCE AMONG PRACTITIONERS AND PATIENTS ABOUT THE USE OF POWER

There is always, inevitably, a power differential when one person with a particular need comes for help from someone who is, or is seen to be, more knowledgeable and more skilled. Many practitioners feel uncomfortable about acknowledging this difference in power between themselves and their patients. On the one hand, the desire to be liked by one's patients and to appear as a warm, caring, compassionate healer can lead to a pretence that there is little or no difference between the patient and practitioner. In this case, the practitioner's skill, expertise and knowledge may be underplayed and underused. On the other hand, particularly for those practitioners who rely greatly on their technical competence, power may be so taken for granted that they do not consciously realize that they have it. Rollo May, in his book *Power and innocence*, suggests that in our culture, 'Power is widely coveted and rarely admitted. Generally, those who have power repress their awareness of this fact' (May 1972: 14). In this case, there is a danger that the patient's vulnerability in relation to the practitioner may be forgotten, so that he may feel that his needs are disregarded or, at worst, that he may be exploited or abused within the therapeutic relationship.

Practitioners tread delicately on a tightrope between, on the one hand, trying to ensure that insofar as they have power and authority it is used humanely and wisely to aid the patient's recovery and, on the other hand, not rendering the patient passive and impotent in the face of the practitioner's competence.

Practitioners have reason to be aware of their potential power and yet also to recoil from this knowledge; in any case, most practitioners probably feel themselves to be less powerful than their patients might sometimes wish them to be. To the extent that they may succeed in persuading patients to follow their advice, and in so doing help patients to combat disease, recover from illness or cope with sickness, therapists have direct opportunities to experience their own effectiveness (and hence power) as healers. However, in the face of intractable distress and suffering and the eventual inevitability of death, practitioners are also frequently brought face to face with their own impotence. They simply cannot be as powerful as patients may sometimes wish them to be.

Patients may have magical hopes that physicians could be powerful enough to ward off illness and even death itself. It seems possible that, ironically, much dissatisfaction with conventional medicine stems from its success in dealing with many illnesses: if it can do so much, even more may be dreamed of in the way of conquering suffering yet, disappointingly, the returns seem to be diminishing. Moreover, in the face of the success of scientific knowledge, skill and technology, people are often left feeling personally and spiritually diminished: powerless, helpless, ineffective and insignificant. When ill, patients want and need the therapists' skill and authority and indeed, the use of skill in the correct application of the appropriate technique may often be just what is needed to deal with the disease. Yet if the therapist can also use her authority to help the patient establish or regain his own sense of personal power and control, then there is likely to be a greater chance of also successfully managing the illness and sickness.

DEFINITIONS OF POWER

There is an important distinction, in considering the meaning of power, between internal and external power. Dictionary definitions of the word 'power' (which stems from the Latin root *posse*, meaning 'to be able') imply both internal and external power: the power to do or effect something in and of oneself, and power and authority over someone else. Two definitions in the *Oxford English Dictionary* which convey these different meanings are:

- ability to act or affect something strongly; physical or mental strength; might; vigour; energy; force of character; telling force; effect
- possession of control or command over others; dominion, rule; government, domination, sway, command; control, influence, authority.

A long-standing issue in medicine is that healing has been viewed as requiring *either* the use of external force on behalf of the patient (as in the tradition of Asclepius) *or* the mobilization of the patient's own internal healing resources or power (as in the Hygeian tradition). Perhaps the most effective healing does both: it may not be a question of either internal or external power but rather, how can the power of the practitioner and of the patient most effectively be brought together?

THE NEED FOR PRACTITIONER AUTHORITY

In his book *The way of the physician*, Needleman (1985) expressed his belief in the importance of the *authority* of the physician, which he contrasted with *authoritarianism* which simply encourages passivity on the part of the patient. Needleman differentiated between two kinds of illness: one that is mainly a mechanical disturbance needing mechanical repair and the other that requires inner 'psychic power' on the part of the sick person, where psychic power is the individual's personal ability to heal, based on his sense of meaning in life, motivation, determination and will-power. In some ways this differentiation corresponds to that made in Chapter 2 between disease and illness, where disease involves the idea of something structurally or function-ally wrong with the person's body (a mechanical disturbance), while illness is a more complex interplay between disease and the person's own subjective experience within a cultural context. Needleman suggested that the success of modern medical tech-nology in dealing with the more mechanical illnesses (or diseases) has led to a neglect of the need to strengthen the patient's own inner will when dealing with more complex illnesses.

Needleman felt that the exercise of personal authority on the part of the physician is necessary in order to strengthen the will of the patient. His point was that, in illness, all one's psychic energy is absorbed by bodily functions, so external help is often needed in order to free some of this energy for self-attention. The authority of the practitioner facilitates the shift of energy into a personal will to overcome the illness. We would develop Needleman's notion to explore further the stages of healing. Especially in the early or acute stages of illness, energy needs to be directed to bodily functions: when physically and emotionally depleted, the patient needs to trust that his physician can take charge. The practitioner's skill lies in judging when to let go of her authority to allow the individual to take over the healing process once he has regathered his own resources.

Needleman is careful to point out that it should not be thought that encouraging inner strength is somehow less real than direct physical treatment. He felt that in this modern era, we have lost our understanding of the deep reality of human attention or will and we mask our ignorance through use of the term 'psychosomatic'. But he was also suspicious of potential charlatans, and stressed that we must not encourage a sort of fantasy of inner will rather than its reality, and especially must not rely on fantasy when physical or technical means are really what is needed. In other words, physical or technical means must be used in treating disease when they are appropriate and, in helping deal with illness, there should be an authentic effort to strengthen the patient's real, inner strength through conveying a belief in his psychic power.

EROSION OF MEDICAL AUTHORITY

The views expressed by Needleman resonate with much of what is written by complementary practitioners about the fundamental need to facilitate the patient's own healing potential and it is very helpful to consider that this may be done through the therapeutic relationship as well as through more technical means. In part, the power and authority of the medical practitioner comes through the social legitimization of her role as healer. To this extent, she is powerful because her expertise has been socially sanctioned (Friedson 1970). The doctor may effectively control the consultation process, being empowered to diagnose and treat disease and to legitimate the claim of the patient to sickness. Patients may be expected to comply with medical advice. Yet, in recent years, the authority of physicians has been much eroded. Social science has recovered the patient as a person who also has a point of view (Radley 1994). Some patients, perhaps particularly exemplified by those who are moving to complementary practitioners, are looking for more equal healing relationships.

The erosion of medical authority is an enormously complex issue: the move to a more egalitarian society is associated with a challenge to professionalism in many spheres of life. Specifically with regard to medicine, sociological and psychological critiques have brought to light the impact of the power of the doctor and the consequent costs to society and the individual in terms of loss of freedom and choice. On the other hand, challenges to professionalism, through the reduced appreciation of the role of the professional in society, have tended to erode the personal satisfaction that doctors and practitioners may derive from their work (Jacob 1988).

At a social level, two influential critics have been the moral philosopher and theologian Ivan Illich and the Marxist socio-logist Lesley Doyal. Ivan Illich, in his book *Medical nemesis* (1975), began the documentation of the ill effects of medicine (iatrogenesis), of which the most important for our purposes was what he called structural iatrogenesis. This referred to the loss of people's ability to take responsibility for their own self-care. The rise in the medical monopoly of control over health care (and its support by the drug industry) in the 19th century, continuing into the 20th century, has been documented by medical sociologists and geographers (Jones & Moon 1987). Twentieth-century scientific medicine was seen as focusing on specialist knowledge which removed the relevance of the judgement of ordinary people and thus reduced the role of the patient, and his social and family network, in managing his day-to-day health care.

Illich, among others, believed that the increased dependence of patients on the technical skill of medical experts led to a loss in capacity to take care of themselves. He favoured deprofessionalization, removing the licensing and regulation of medical practitioners so as to leave people free to enter health care relationships with whomever they chose. In the light of Illich's criticism it is apposite to note the move towards increased regulation of the complementary health professions.

On the whole, patients who come to complementary practitioners seem to have particular health beliefs which lead them to wish for and to value more egalitarian relationships with practitioners. Stone & Matthews (1996) question whether, given the change in role of the patient in complementary practice compared to orthodox practice, holistic medicine is actually capable of being formally regulated in any meaningful way. They contrast the orthodox doctor–patient relationship, in which the doctor is the expert and the patient the passive recipient of treatment, with a relationship based on mutual responsibilities and commitment in which information, and thus power, is shared. Ironically, the orthodox medico-legal model of regulation (although ostensibly intended to protect patients' interests) may well be damaging to patient autonomy, since it carries with it an implication that patients have a passive rather than an active position within the therapeutic relationship.

At a sociopolitical level, it would seem that all powerful groups have a vested interest in maintaining their own dominance. Through attempting to adopt statutory regulatory frameworks, complementary practitioners seem to be moving towards greater power in society. In opposition to this, Stone & Matthews call for a patient-centred, non-statutory regulatory framework with clear systems for registration, a strong code of ethics and effective and accessible grievance procedures. They argue that such a model acknowledges patients of complementary practitioners as autonomous agents, capable of making personal choices and with obligations to play an active part in treatment.

Doyal & Pennell, in *The political economy of health* (1979), rejected Illich's focus on individual self-help. They asserted that structural inequalities in society mean that relatively disadvantaged individuals have little choice about their lifestyles (whether it be amount of exercise, housing conditions, diet or consumption of cigarettes) which may be associated with poor health. They favoured a 'demand for a radically different socioeconomic order', along with equality of access to medical care and demystification of medical knowledge.

It is the case that many modern-day patients want to assert their power in relation to health care professionals and to take some control in the management of illness. Sociological and psychological analyses of the doctor–patient relationship have appeared in the media and patients are becoming aware that in some ways they have been disadvantaged by doctors' powers over them. For example, in a newspaper article in *The Independent* (June 1995), patients were urged to give their doctors a hard time by becoming more assertive. It was claimed that research had shown that enlightened, assertive patients manage chronic illness and its associated stresses more effectively.

Haug (1988) documented the rise of the new consumerism since the 1960s: increasingly some (not all) patients wish to take an active part in sharing information, in decision making, in treatment and in self-care. The political movement towards consumerism is enshrined in influential policy documents such as *The Patient's Charter* which purport to empower patients within the health care market place. The consumerist model potentially shifts the balance of power between patient and practitioner, since it is based on the economic power of the patient as purchaser of a service (either directly through his own pocket or through his influence on the resources of the purchasing health commission or fund-holding GP). In this context, complementary medicine is coming to be seen as the treatment of choice for those patients who have the economic power to sustain their informed decisions about their own health care.

OMNIPOTENCE AND VULNERABILITY

There is a risk that practitioners' power in relation to patients may go too far, since dominant social groups are apt to protect their privileges and status through the control of knowledge and information. If the practitioner believes that she knows best, this can be at the expense of what the patient himself knows. Masson (1992), in his book *Against therapy*, produced a damning critique of the power relation between patient and practitioner in the case of psychotherapy. In the book's preface, the psychologist Dorothy Rowe defined power as 'the right to have your definition of reality prevail over all other people's definition of reality' (Rowe, in Masson 1992: 16). She went on to argue:

Many people who wish to impose their definition of reality would deny that they are involved in gaining power. They would say that because of their greater knowledge, wisdom, training and experience they know what is best. The most dangerous people in the world are those who believe that they know what is best for others. (Rowe, in Masson 1992: 17)

Such people do not question their own prejudices; indeed, they are unlikely to become aware that they have prejudices since they can take their own truth for granted. Unfortunately, in doing so they run the risk of denying other people's truth. This issue is very problematic in health care since, at least at a technical level, there are times, as Needleman asserts, when the patient needs the practitioner to know best. Any 'knowing best' must always be a temporary state of affairs, framed in the context of the recognition of practitioners' and patients' common humanity, shared vulnerability and potential fallibility. The real danger comes when the practitioner and patient collude in the belief that the practitioner is, in all cases and at all times, omnipotent.

Various writers who have considered the psychological aspects of the power relationship between practitioner and patient have noted this tendency towards omnipotence on the part of the practitioner. Bourne (1981), in the book *Under the doctor* which examines the psychological problems of physiotherapists, patients and doctors, noted that anyone who treats illness is under pressure to behave as if omnipotent. Bennet (1987), in *The wound and the doctor*, identified the grand manner, perpetual business and impersonal behaviour (all the trappings of authority and success) as strategies which allow the doctor to avoid the disturbing effects of patients' distress:

He is not real to his patients because they perceive no evidence of a genuine person. He gives them nothing but his expertise – which may be very well worth having on its own – and he remains untouched. (Bennet 1987: 167)

There is no reason why complementary practitioners (or indeed any other health professional) should be immune from this pressure towards omnipotence. The Jungian psychoanalyst Adolph Guggenbühl-Craig (1971) tried to analyse this question of power for all helping professionals. He used Jung's concept of the archetype: a hypothetical inborn potential of behaviour common to everyone. People are considered to react archetypally when faced with a typical relationship which constantly recurs in the human condition, such as parent–child, teacher–pupil, male–female, doctor–patient. In Jung's view, each archetype has two poles which are inherently contained within one individual but, because of our human discomfort with the tension of ambivalence, are inclined to be split between individuals who interact together. In the case of the doctor–patient archetype, when a person becomes ill or when a person becomes a practitioner, the doctor–patient archetype is activated, but the tendency is for one person to become 'only a patient' and the other to become 'only a doctor'. Yet, Guggenbühl-Craig argued, what is needed for true healing to take place is for the inner healer to be activated in the patient and, reciprocally, the inner patient to be activated in the healer (Guggenbühl-Craig 1971).

The danger comes when the practitioner assumes all the power of being the healer; she can surround herself with the trappings of power, with the sense that only she can facilitate the cure, while the patient can sit back and rely completely on the practitioner. The practitioner may thus push away any awareness of her own vulnerability or weakness; she sees sickness only in the patient who may be degraded and denied the possibility of activating his own power in terms of dealing with his illness. Guggenbühl-Craig asserted that those who have a vocation for becoming a practitioner have a particular fascination with the doctor–patient archetype, for a variety of psychological reasons which have subsequently been documented by Bennet (1987), among others (see Ch. 9). In Bennet's view, only those practitioners who are able to accept vulnerability and sickness as existential possibilities for themselves can become true 'wounded healers' whose patients can then be freed to use their own healing capacity.

CONSTRUCTIVE USE OF POWER

Why *do* people listen to, and sometimes even act on, the advice of practitioners? Anthropological and sociopsychological evidence suggests that it is, in part, the socially sanctioned status of the practitioner (in traditional healing, psychotherapy, counselling and modern medicine) which mobilizes the hope and expectancy of the patient and inclines him to do as the practitioner suggests (Kleinman & Sung 1979). Frank, in *Persuasion and healing* (1973), was the first to make explicit the idea that the healer can use her power to persuade the patient towards more effective coping. Various psychological writers, notably Strong & Claiborn (1982), have subsequently elaborated his ideas, drawing too on the notions of social power put forward by sociologists such as French & Raven (1959). Strong & Claiborn see treatment or therapy as a form of social influence in which one person, the patient, because of his dependence on the resources of another, the practitioner, will change himself in accordance with the practitioner's demands; in other words, he will do as the practitioner expects. However, if this is to happen in a constructive way, the practitioner must have resources (skills, knowledge and experience) which are genuine and relevant and she must be a person who does care about the well-being of the other.

The therapeutic task is to convey a sense of mastery, of having a belief in the possibility of personal control over internal responses and relevant external circumstances. In Needleman's terms, this is what is meant by strengthening the patient's will.

POWER WITHIN SOCIAL INFLUENCE THEORY

Another way of conceptualizing power issues is provided by Strong & Claiborn (1982), who argued that the practitioner influences the patient through her social power. Schaap et al (1993) identified several power bases which make up social power, each of which refers to a relationship between a particular need of the patient and a particular quality of the practitioner. For the purposes of our discussion, two of these power bases are particularly relevant to the treatment aims in complementary therapies: expert power and referent power.

Expert power

This is based on the relationship between the practitioner's knowledge, skills and experience and the patient's need for specialized help in managing his problems. Expert power is invoked when the practitioner's external power is used on the patient's behalf, in terms of directly challenging the disease or illness. A patient will be inclined to engage with the practitioner in treatment and to trust and follow her advice to the extent that he is convinced of her expertise. Recognition of the practitioner's expertise comes through three main sources: technical competence, social validation (formal recognition of training and status) and reputation.

Referent power

This is based on the relationship between the practitioner's personal resources and the patient's need to have someone with whom he can realistically compare himself and whose positive qualities he can aspire to and wish to integrate into his own sense of self. Referent power is invoked when the practitioner attempts to strengthen the patient's own internal power and capacity to heal himself.

We can separate out three aspects of referent power: the recognized conditions for therapeutic effectiveness, which are warmth, empathy and genuineness (Rogers 1951); being a real person with weaknesses as well as strengths; and attribution of success to the patient's own capacities.

MISUSE OF POWER: SEXUAL ABUSE IN THERAPY

Perhaps the most obvious and extreme form of the exploitation of power in the therapeutic relationship is that which occurs when patient and practitioner become sexually intimate. While sexual abuse within therapy remains, as far as we know, a relatively rare event, it could be considered the 'tip of the iceberg' of wider and more general abuse within treatment. For that reason, it is worth enlarging on some of what is known about such abuse in the hope that this may shed some light on more common, though perhaps less extreme, distortions in the balance of power in the therapeutic relationship.

In his book *Patients as victims*, Jehu (1994) reviewed the adverse consequences for patients following sexual involvement with their therapists in psychotherapy and counselling, and discussed what may be done to avoid abuse and to intervene when abuse has taken place. Much of this section is drawn from Jehu's scholarly book; there are no publications yet available which discuss this issue within complementary health treatment and so we must learn what we can from knowledge of related therapies. The (limited) evidence which is available accords with beliefs enshrined in all medical ethical traditions: patients who become sexually involved with practitioners are likely to suffer harm. The establishment of sexual intimacy with a therapist is often a traumatic event which is psychologically distressing to the patient. The harm relates to the breach of trust experienced by the patient, who feels a profound sense of helplessness (the opposite of the enhancement of morale and effectiveness which should be engendered in effective treatment).

Jehu stressed that because of the power differential between therapists and patients, therapists hold all the ethical responsibility for their actions: patients cannot be held to blame since they are dependent on the practitioner for help. Jehu summarized the reasons for the universal prohibition of sexual activity in therapeutic settings (while noting that sexual attraction may be statistically normal and to be expected to occur sometimes; it is acting on the attraction which is harmful). The reasons for avoiding sexual intimacy are: breach of trust; violation of the professional role; exploitation of the patient's vulnerability; misuse of power; absence of consent; impairment of the therapeutic process; negative consequences for the patient; and disrepute of the profession.

Factors associated with sexual abuse in treatment

Therapist factors

Sexual misconduct has been found to be more common in practitioners who tend to behave in generally dominating or antisocial ways, who may be experiencing personal distress or professional isolation, who use drugs or alcohol or rationalizations to overcome any inhibitions they may feel and who attempt to persuade patients by breaking normal boundary rules or who use the therapeutic relationship as leverage towards increasing intimacy.

Patient factors

All patients are to some extent dependent on the person whom they have consulted for help, but more excessively dependent patients are at particular risk of exploitation (especially those who have a history of previously being abused). Such patients may be convinced of their own helplessness and feel the need for someone to rely on; consequently they may overidealize the practitioner. Alternatively, some patients may assume a sense of responsibility and care for the practitioner and thereby open themselves to becoming too close and intimate.

POWER IN TREATMENT: IMPLICATIONS FOR PRACTICE

Keeping track of the power relationship in treatment, and considering what action might avoid the power relationship becoming distorted, requires self-regulation on the part of the practitioner. The practitioner needs to monitor carefully her own thoughts, feelings and behaviour in relation to patients. Noting warning signs and acting on them in advance can help to ensure that no harm befalls patients in treatment. Jehu suggested that four factors are necessary preconditions for sexual abuse to occur: therapist motivation; breakdown of internal inhibitions; lack of external constraints; and the patient's lack of power. These factors can be used as a more general framework for considering the balance of power in all therapeutic relationships.

Clarify personal motivation: keep power in perspective

- Explore your reasons for becoming a practitioner through supervision, guided reflection or personal therapeutic work (see also Ch. 9).
- Be careful to ensure that patients' needs take precedence over your own.
- Take responsibility for ensuring that your own needs to be caring and to be intimate are met in other places as well as in your consulting room.
- Be especially careful to get personal support during times of stress and distress.

Maintain appropriate internal inhibitions

Develop an awareness of the process of transference and countertransference. Remember that the patient's transference of powerful feelings (both negative and positive) from previous important relationships can push and flatter the practitioner into feeling more significant and powerful than is appropriate. A dangerous countertransference can be the belief that only the practitioner can 'save' the patient, leading to more and more 'heroic' efforts to help and to take over the patient's life.

1. Be sensitive to your own thoughts, feelings and behaviour towards individual patients before, during and after treatment sessions. Warning signs of potential problems include:

- feelings of irritation, anger or resentment towards patients
- making exceptions to your usual rules about treatment boundaries
- a tendency to blame or criticize patients
- finding yourself beginning to think of particular patients as 'types' rather than individuals (depersonalizing patients).

2. Check whether you are able to 'switch off' after treatment sessions. Warning signs of not being able to do so include:

- intrusive thoughts about treatment issues
- frequent dreams about patients
- inability to enjoy relaxation and leisure.

3. Monitor your ability to allow patients' expression of emotions.

- An avoidance of intense emotion can come across as rigid and impersonal.
- Conversely, too much pushing for emotional expression may be experienced as intrusive and inappropriate.
- Enable patients to feel free to choose how much emotion to express and when to do so.

4. Check on who does most of the talking in treatment sessions: too much talking on your part can overpower the patient. Keep the balance by ensuring that you:

- ask plenty of open questions
- clarify details with closed questions
- only express your views and opinions in the context of the patient's own understanding.

Establish external constraints

The practitioner should be sensitive to patients' experiences of vulnerability: the more the patient feels vulnerable, fears abandonment and lacks a sense of self-identity and self-esteem, the greater is the risk that the practitioner will inappropriately take charge and thereby perpetuate the patient's difficulties. Therefore, clear boundaries need to be set in order to avoid too much intrusion into the patient's life.

- Find ways of getting support, advice and supervision from colleagues, both as a matter of routine and for consultation over difficult or problematic situations.
- Establish clear expectations about length, frequency and place of consultation and do not change these for individual patients without careful thought and explanation.
- Be realistic about what can and cannot be expected to be achieved in treatment and convey these expectations honestly to patients.
- Recognize that it is not possible for anyone, practitioner or patient, to have ultimate control over what happens within a relationship. When things go wrong, sometimes ending or transferring to another practitioner may be the best solution, as long as this is done with care, tact and sensitivity.
- Read, understand and follow your profession's ethical guidelines and codes of conduct.
- Make sure that patients know how, and to whom, to complain if things go wrong (information on making complaints should be displayed in every waiting room).

Enhance patients' power

This final section brings us back to the central theme of treatment as facilitation of the patient's own healing resources. The facilitative practitioner aims to use her power to help the patient to find his own ways of dealing with his illness. She therefore does all she can to establish and enhance the patient's own sense of control and mastery. This requires the collaborative approach to treatment which is implicit throughout this book.

- Find out as much as you can from patients about what they want from treatment.
- Wherever possible, decide together with patients about aims for treatment and care.
- Agree with patients about how to monitor and evaluate treatment.

- Do all you can to enter the patient's world and to see things from his perspective, especially during those periods of treatment when you need to be more actively authoritative.
- Encourage patients' choices by carefully and adequately explaining your treatment approach and making it possible for patients to consent *or* withdraw from treatment without embarrassment, loss of face or fear of disappointing you.
- Give plenty of opportunity for patients to ask questions.
- Recognize and acknowledge the patient's part in any successful treatment.

REFERENCES

Bennet G 1987 The wound and the doctor. Secker and Warburg, London
Bourne S 1981 Under the doctor. Avebury, Amersham
Doyal L, Pennell I 1979 The political economy of health. Pluto Press, London
Frank J D 1973 Persuasion and healing, 2nd edn. Johns Hopkins University Press, Baltimore
French J R P, Raven B 1959 The bases of social power. In: Cartwright D (ed) Studies in social power. University of Michigan Press, Ann Arbor
Friedson E (1970) Profession of medicine. Dodd, Mead, New York
Guggenbühl-Craig A 1971 Power in the helping profession. Spring, Dallas
Haug M R 1988 Power, authority and health behaviour. In: Gochman D S (ed) Health behavior: emerging research perspectives. Plenum Press, New York, pp 325–336
Illich I 1975 Medical nemesis. Calder and Boyars, London
Jacob J M 1988 Doctors and rules: a sociology of professional values. Routledge, London
Jehu D 1994 Patients as victims. Sexual abuse in psychotherapy and counselling. Wiley, Chichester
Jones K, Moon G 1987 Health, disease and society: an introduction to medical geography. Routledge, London
Kleinman A, Sung L H 1979 Why do indigenous practitioners successfully heal? Social Science and Medicine 138:7–26
May R 1972 Power and innocence. W W Norton, New York
Masson J 1992 Against therapy. Fontana, London
Needleman J 1985 The way of the physician. Penguin, Harmondsworth
Radley A 1994 Making sense of illness: the social psychology of health and disease. Sage, London
Rogers C R 1951 Client-centred therapy. Constable, London
Schaap C, Bennun I, Schindler L, Hoogduin K 1993 The therapeutic relationship in behavioural psychotherapy. Wiley, Chichester
Stone J, Matthews J 1996 Complementary medicine and the law. Oxford University Press, Oxford
Strong S S, Claiborn C D 1982 Change through interaction. Wiley, New York

8

The process of treatment

In this chapter, we set out a model of the treatment process to provide a framework for practitioners to develop therapeutic relationships with their patients which are in harmony with their broader therapeutic endeavours. An emphasis on enhancing self-healing means working in a way which facilitates patients' healthy development since, as discussed in Chapter 2, there is a parallel between the idea of self-healing capacity and development. Many practitioners will be concerned with empowering their patients: trying to give them confidence to play a part in controlling their illness.

A DEVELOPMENTAL CONTEXT FOR TREATMENT

Accounts of the process of treatment in the psychotherapy literature draw a parallel between the developmental experiences of the child and the therapeutic experiences of the adult. Howe (1993) argued that it is no surprise that the troubled adult emphasizes the quality of the relationship with the practitioner when seeking help, since it is through the experience of relationships with others that development takes place. The works of developmental psychologists (e.g. Bowlby 1969, Richards 1974, Richards & Light 1986), social psychologists (e.g. Mead 1934) and philosophers (Berger & Luckman 1966) emphasized the social nature of the self: they postulated that the self arises through relationships with others.

The developing child is immersed from birth in a world of relationships; attachments to others are formed out of, and form the basis for, interactive dialogue and communication, through which the child discovers that he and others have thoughts, feelings and intentions and can be active in dealing with the world. When interactions with others are reliable, predictable and enjoyable he experiences a sense of security and trust out of which can arise feelings of confidence, competence and positive self-esteem.

It is suggested that, in order to combat the demoralization associated with illness, the adult sufferer needs a therapeutic relationship which parallels the relationship between the infant and caregiver in which he feels secure and cared for. Howe put it like this:

... if it can be argued that self, identity, personality and the basis of understanding are formed within a matrix of social relationships, it will not be a surprise to learn that those who are experiencing personal and interpersonal problems seek a return to the kind of social relationship in which the self originally formed. This is not regression in the sense that an individual is returning to immature ways of coping. The structures and processing characteristics of the brain, having formed in relationship with others, are then precisely equipped to make sense of those kind of relationships and the experiences that arise within them. (Howe 1993: 13)

When the troubled person experiences a mixture of somatic symptoms and psychological distress (as seems to be the case for most illness; see Ch. 1), then pain, discomfort, malaise and fatigue may lead the patient both to need and to want to relinquish ordinary day-to-day responsibilities and to depend on others for care. Disease, illness and the sick role all emphasize the individual's vulnerability and dependence and therefore may all be associated with 'regression' to a more childlike position in relation to others. Frank (1973) noted how patients who are ill and faced with un-successful efforts to deal with threat inevitably fall back on patterns of behaviour that they developed in early life to cope with similar predicaments. It seems important, then, that the process of treatment includes a phase which allows for the patient's dependency and which gives the patient a sense of protection and safety. This provides a secure base for those aspects of treatment which are about challenging and dealing with symptoms.

In his review of psychotherapy clients' views of treatment, Howe (1993) identified three themes which characterized experiences of the therapeutic sequence. He argued that these themes, 'accept me', 'understand me' and 'talk with me', echo three major areas of psychological and social development in childhood:

- *attachment*: the establishment of a secure emotional base in which the person feels accepted and safe
- *understanding*: making sense of people and relationships
- *language*: the development of a shared framework for communicating meaning and understanding.

Howe saw the treatment process as having three phases which relate to these developmental themes in childhood.

1. The client becomes immersed in a relationship with another person. If treatment is to be successful, this relationship needs to be one in which the client feels himself to be liked and accepted by a warm and friendly practitioner. This provides the secure base for treatment.
2. The client and practitioner together try to understand the meaning of the client's experiences.
3. By making sense of what has happened, the client may wish to go on to develop new ways of looking at what is happening and possibly to generate more appropriate ways of coping.

In a different account of the therapeutic process, Skynner (1986) used the metaphor of the parent–child relationship, where the patient is seen as the child and the practitioner as the parent. Skynner's summary of the developmental sequence in childhood is:

- an initial, highly dependent, infantile relationship
- a struggle for independence and autonomy (characterized by rebelliousness and anger)
- a concern for establishing equal and mutual relationships.

Skynner saw the process of development being re-enacted in therapy and he argued that the therapist's role at each point needs to be appropriate to the stage which the treatment is recapitulating. Thus, in the early stages, where dependency is to the fore, the practitioner may be idealized and needs to be supportive, nurturing and not to show negative feelings and failures. In the middle stages of struggle for autonomy, the emphasis for the therapist will be on holding firm in terms of structure, being more robust, assertive and, perhaps, confrontational; in other words, more challenging. In the later stages, moving towards equality and mutuality, the therapist needs to be more open, equal, transparent, personal and human, with an element of lightheartedness.

Benefits and limitations of the developmental approach

Developmental accounts of the therapeutic process may provide a useful framework for conceptualizing clients' or patients' changing needs as treatment proceeds. The parental metaphor is useful insofar as treatment is seen as a way of helping the patient to move from a dependent to a more independent position vis-à-vis his illness *and* in relation to the practitioner.

However, the developmental approach to treatment has two important limitations. The first is based on a concern that too narrow a focus on the individual within the therapeutic relationship draws attention away from the broader social context of disease, illness and sickness. The second limitation is to do with the reality of the therapeutic relationship which is actually (with adult patients) a relationship between two adults, not between an adult and child.

The need for complementary practitioners to be aware of the broader social context of illness

Part of the underpinning for the application of most complementary approaches is the concept of holism, with its emphasis on the integration of the whole system of mind, body and spirit. Yet, as Rosalind Coward (1989) pointed out, it is ironic that holism, as applied in complementary health treatments, rarely pays little more than lip service to the significance of the wider systems of family and society in which the individual is embedded. She noted that the writings of many complementary practitioners convey the view that the individual holds personal responsibility for his own health and illness. There is a danger that this sense of responsibility may carry over into a conviction that illness is a personal failure on the part of the individual. Smail (1994) suggested that guilt at not being able to solve the individual's problem is something to which many practitioners are prone and which they try to assuage by placing the burden of responsibility onto the patient.

The individualistic emphasis ignores the significance of the well-established evidence that poor health is associated with social inequalities (Townsend & Davidson 1982, Wilkinson 1996). In a review of socioeconomic health inequalities, Carroll et al (1993) concluded that individual factors (such as poor social relations, psychological stress, absence of control) are surface factors, while socioeconomic inequality remains the basic cause of inequalities in health. They warned that interventions focused on the individual could, inadvertently, contribute to victim blaming and may divert attention away from social/political efforts which might directly address inequality.

The implications for an understanding of the process of treatment must be to:

- draw the attention of the practitioner to the wider world in which the patient lives
- see treatment as taking place in a broad social context
- acknowledge those factors which are beyond the control of the individual
- consider ways of empowering the patient within his social world, as well as within the therapeutic relationship.

Dangers of the parental metaphor

While the process of treatment may at times and in part mirror the process of 'growing up', this is only in the context of two experienced people bringing together their different understandings, knowledge and skills to try to solve a problem. If this is ignored, then patients run the risk of being disrespected, patronized, belittled and abused. Since the parental metaphor is dominant in our paternalistic culture, it is easy to see the risk of the patient being maintained in a position where 'parent' (doctor, therapist, practitioner) knows best and where his own knowledge and skills are underplayed.

Laypeople always stand in danger of being disempowered by expert professionals, to the extent that the professionals' claim to expertise is through their ownership of technical skills and expert knowledge which are seen as superior to (as well as different from) the skills and knowledge of the layperson. Complementary practitioners (their emphasis on the patient's own healing power notwithstanding) run as much risk of treating their patients this way as more orthodox practitioners, especially if complementary medicine continues its current move towards more regulated professional status. This risk may be reduced by an emphasis on the importance of the therapeutic relationship relative to the use of skills and knowledge, but only if the relationship is one which recognizes the fundamental mutuality of the participants.

TREATMENT AS A PROCESS OF SOCIAL INFLUENCE

In Chapter 6, we looked at the theoretical and empirical bases for understanding treatment as a process of social influence. It was seen that the practitioner's expert and referent powers can be used by patients as resources to combat the demoralization associated with illness (Schaap et al 1993). In trying to develop a model of the process of treatment, it is important to consider how the power relationship between the practitioner and patient may need to change over time. During the course of treatment there is likely to be a shift in the balance of power between patient and practitioner and a shift in the use of sources of power within the therapeutic relationship. This will be taken into account below in considering the model of the treatment process.

TOWARDS A MODEL OF THE THERAPEUTIC PROCESS

A useful model of the therapeutic process should take into account the central tension in treatment, summed up in Freud's famous phrase *Lieben und arbeiten* (to love and to work), which draws attention to the distinction, found in most accounts of the nature of healing, of the two dimensions of *care* and *challenge*.

The first dimension, *care*, is to do with the 'art' of healing: here the practitioner's intuition, creativity and wisdom are emphasized, together with her compassion and capacity to relate sensitively to and to provide care for her patients. In the terms of social influence theory, this is where the practitioner uses referent power. The second dimension, *challenge*, is to do with the 'science' of healing: the use of techniques and knowledge in challenging the symptoms of disease and illness. To the fore here are the practitioner's technical skills and rational understanding, together with her strength, decisiveness, resilience and capacity to exercise her personal authority. Again, in terms of social influence theory, this dimension involves the use of expert power.

The split between 'art' and 'science' has a parallel in our knowledge about the different aspects of mental functioning which have been related to the left and right sides of the brain. Right hemisphere function, in most people, is associated with more intuitive, imaginative, symbolic activity, while the left hemisphere is more involved with rational, verbal, logical thought (Sperry et al 1969).

By and large, our Western society tends to value (some may say to overvalue) the technical successes associated with left hemisphere activity. Thus, as Watts (1992) pointed out, Western orthodox medicine is seen to have based its technical success on the rational use of reductionist scientific principles yet, in doing so, it has embraced science almost to the exclusion of all else, so that the personal significance of the therapeutic encounter has been largely lost. In orthodox medicine, technology is primary, while personal experience is relegated to the background. The revival of interest in complementary medicine, insofar as it relies relatively less on technology and more on personal meaning, can be seen as part of a shift away from the emphasis on rationality, science and technology.

It seems, in practice, to be difficult to hold a balance between 'art' and 'science' or between 'love' and 'work'. We tend to slip in one direction or the other. Yet, as Needleman (1985) pointed out, these two aspects of healing must be held together. He saw the authentic physician as both a healer and a person of knowledge who holds two kinds of power: a strong life energy and a well-developed intellect. Life energy should be used with a good background knowledge, otherwise it may produce haphazard results or cause more harm than good. Intellect without life energy cannot directly affect the patient's self-healing forces and may therefore only lead to temporary and perhaps superficial results in treatment and then only for those patients with acute rather than chronic illnesses.

The point here is that both intellect and life energy are necessary but, perhaps, at different points in the therapeutic process. Part of the value of a model of the process of treatment is to provide a context for understanding when the different styles are needed.

Benefits of using a model of the process of treatment

A model of the process of treatment should provide a framework to enable practitioners to:

- see treatment within the context of the patient's real life, which includes their familial, social and cultural network

- provide a balance between the more rational, technical 'work' aspects and the more intuitive, personal 'love' aspects of treatment
- think carefully about power in the therapeutic relationship
- build up therapeutic relationships which are productive, which can facilitate healing and which can end appropriately
- treat the person's own subjective experience of his disorder: that is, treat *illness*, not just disease
- identify the less immediately obvious aspects of treatment so that the patient's changing needs can be attended to throughout treatment
- identify what might be going wrong when treatment seems not to be progressing and what may need to be done to get things moving again
- actively use the placebo or non-specific aspects of treatment as integral components of a holistic approach.

A MODEL OF THE PROCESS OF TREATMENT

The model summarizes those aspects of treatment which have been seen to be important and puts them together in a sequential order. The order of events in treatment is not invariant, but there is usually an emphasis on one aspect of treatment rather than another at any one point in time. Each phase in the process is seen not as an isolated, unconnected event but rather within the context of the requirements of all the other aspects of treatment.

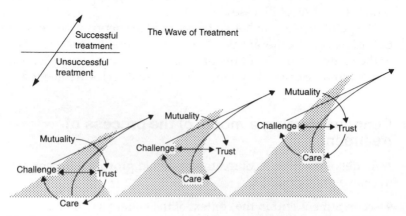

Fig. 2 The process of treatment (reproduced with permission from Mitchell 1995).

The model is best conceptualized as a spiral or series of waves, allowing for the possibility of upward movement (improvement) and downward movement (deterioration). (Any therapeutic act has the potential for harm as well as benefit.) The outcome of certain phases of treatment may enhance or diminish the impact of other phases. The model is illustrated, in diagrammatic form, in Figure 2.

The phases of treatment

Phase 1   Mutuality: a foundation of mutual respect, positive expectations coupled with recognition of limits and shared understanding

Phase 2   Trust: the provision of containment, security and safety within the therapeutic relationship and in the treatment setting

Phase 3   Care: the experience of a caring, accepting therapeutic relationship

Phase 4   Challenge: the practitioner's application of technical skills

Phase 5   Return to mutuality: a more balanced relationship with an agreement for shared responsibilities for future health care, including actions which the patient needs to take for convalescence, self-care and prevention of future illness.

In this model, the more rational, technical, 'work' aspects of treatment are found in the phases of mutuality and challenge (where the emphasis is on making sense, using techniques and practical action). The more intuitive, personal, 'love' aspects are found in the phases of trust and care (where the emphasis is on providing safety and a caring relationship).

Phase 1   Mutuality

At the beginning of treatment, the practitioner and patient need to establish a working alliance based on mutual respect, positive expectations and recognition of limits and an attempt to reach a shared understanding.

Mutual respect

At its simplest, mutual respect means the patient and practitioner behaving towards one another in a frank, polite, straightforward way as ordinary people. For some patients it will require almost heroic efforts simply to cross the threshold to reach the practitioner who therefore should do her best to help them feel welcome and at ease. If the practitioner appears as a credible figure, both competent and friendly, this may mobilize the patient's hope for success. However, if at this point in treatment the practitioner seems too obviously expert and authoritative, then this may reduce the possibility of reaching a genuinely shared under-standing of the patient's difficulties: the patient may feel too much in awe of the practitioner to express things his own way.

Positive expectations and recognition of limits

There is plenty of evidence that the expectations of both prac-titioner and patient influence the outcome of treatment. Positive expectations improve outcome (Richardson 1989; see also Ch. 6). Early in treatment the practitioner needs to convey to the patient her own positive expectations and her own belief in the effec-tiveness of the treatment she uses. Part of the practitioner's task, continuing throughout treatment, is gradually to build up the patient's belief that he can change in the ways needed for effective outcome of treatment (Bandura 1977). Early in the process, this may be based on recognizing the patient as a person who is worthy of time, attention and treatment. Later, it may also mean encouraging, noticing and emphasizing the patient's successes.

On the other hand, expectations should have a realistic basis. It is essential not to hold out false hopes; of course, this is a particular area of concern when working with patients who have life-threatening or terminal conditions. Moreover, it is also necessary to recognize what realistically can and cannot be dealt with in treatment. Some aspects of people's lives which have an impact on their health, such as poverty, employment conditions, poor housing and family circumstances, may be beyond the power of any individual to change. It can come as a relief to patients to have the constraints of their lives acknowledged and taken seriously. Smail wrote:

There is nothing in the least therapeutic in suggesting to people that they can help things they have no influence over, nor is there anything non-therapeutic about clarifying with them that they cannot help things which, indeed, they cannot help ... the demonstration to people that the reasons for their difficulties are beyond their capacity to influence has, in my experience, never been received with anything but relief. (Smail 1994: 8)

As discussed in Chapter 6, rituals can play an important part in healing and their use may be one of the factors which attracts patients to complementary health treatment. 'People are yearning for a richness and meaning to life' (Roose-Evans 1994: 155). Rituals operate at many levels, as Kakar (1982) demonstrated in his book on shamans, mystics and doctors. They can strengthen expectations and hope, can bring in patients as active participants in the process of cure and they can integrate the wider social network, as well as deeper unconscious meanings, into the healing process. Rituals can pull into balance the hopes for change and the realistic constraints on the possibility of change and can open new channels for continued development. Kakar contended:

Basically, the healing rituals seek to connect (or reconnect) the individual with sources of psychological strength available in his or her life situation, and thus counteract the more or less conscious feelings of despair, shame, guilt, inferiority, confusion and isolation in which the 'illness' is embedded. (Kakar 1982: 82)

Shared understanding

During the mutuality phase in treatment, the practitioner takes the patient's history and formulates a diagnosis or conceptualization of the problem on which treatment will be based. On the one hand, the practitioner will be using her expert power, insofar as she will bring to bear her own theoretical or conceptual framework in asking questions and in trying to understand the patient's story. On the other hand, she will use her referent power in helping the patient to tell his own story from his own perspective (Kleinman 1988, Skelton & Groyle 1991). The patient's ideas may be helpful or unhelpful; indeed, as we will see later, it is possible that part of the therapeutic process may be to challenge unproductive ideas. However, this is more likely to happen if, at first, the patient has felt that his ideas have been taken seriously, understood and respected (Tuckett et al 1985).

Early in treatment, then, the practitioner needs to try to enter the patient's conceptual world. It is also important that she conveys her own formulation about the patient's situation in a way which the patient can understand and to pull together her own and the patient's viewpoints in order to reach a shared understanding as a basis for treatment. For some patients, talking through the problem and gaining a new perspective may be enough to move them onwards to tackle the illness in their own way, with no need for further intervention. Others will continue with the treatment process.

Phase 2   Trust

A feeling of safety and containment is the foundation for care and for the patient's willingness to take on the subsequent challenges which may lead to change. Boundaries provide the framework and set the limits for treatment. Clarity about boundaries is important in establishing safety for patients. In addition to the boundary of the treatment setting itself, boundaries include interpersonal factors, such as social taboos, and legal and ethical codes. In particular, respect for confidentiality is of crucial importance. The patient should rightly expect that what is told to the practitioner remains confidential between them unless specific agreement has been given to pass information on to another person. Careful attention needs to be paid to relationships with other professionals who may be dealing with the patient. This is particularly important when the patient is seeing several practitioners or is working simultaneously with orthodox and non-orthodox systems of treatment. In such cases, clarity is needed about who is responsible for which aspects of treatment. Legally, the fundamental provision of safety for patients is incorporated in the duty of care held by all health care workers towards patients to take 'reasonable care in all circumstances' and the *tort of negligence* requiring practitioners to recognize and observe the limits of their professional training and competence.

Temporal boundaries are also of significance here: that is, attention to time in relation to treatment. It is helpful to patients to have an idea of how long treatment is likely to last (individual sessions and course of treatment) and to know whether, how and under what circumstances they can have access to the practitioner outside treatment times or after treatment has ended. If enough care is taken to create clear boundaries, then the therapeutic relationship may become a safe place where the patient can feel relieved of the expectations which pertain in the ordinary encounters elsewhere in his life. He can then become free to try out new ways of being and relating which may be more productive and which may facilitate the changes he needs to make. This is why friendship (social meeting outside the therapeutic context) may impede the change possibilities created by the therapeutic relationship.

Phase 3   Care

During the phase of treatment in which care is to the fore, there is an emphasis on, and concern for, patients' feelings, with a reduction in expert power and an increase in referent power. Frank (1973) suggested that part of the process of combating demoralization is through the patient finding out, within the therapeutic relationship, that the practitioner (even though she may know the 'worst' about him) can feel a sense of positive regard, respect and personal warmth towards him. The warmth conveyed by the practitioner is reminiscent of the symbolism used by the parent who 'kisses it better' for the child. To the extent that the patient respects, trusts and perhaps identifies with the practitioner, he may gain some hope and believe in the value of his efforts to do something to change things or to cope with those things which cannot be changed. Thus, the caring shown by the practitioner may help the patient regain a sense of positive self-regard and personal effectiveness, while at the same time avoid fuelling the propensity for self-blame. Frank (1973) believed that, through the therapeutic relationship, the practitioner supports the patient and provides him with morale-enhancing experiences until he gains the courage to face up to change.

This is the aspect of treatment which patients so often feel to be lacking in orthodox medical care, with its emphasis on technical interventions and rational methods. Patients regret the absence of 'tender loving care'. The important point which patients make is that they wish that professionals would be open enough to really try, at a deep level, to imagine how things feel from the patient's point of view (Consumer Advisory Panel, unpublished report, 1993). However, this is not straightforward. It has been suggested by Bennet (1987) that part of the motivation for becoming a practitioner may be to try to do something about distress as a way of vicariously dealing with the practitioner's own uncomfortable and painful feelings associated with vulnerability. It can be very difficult to acknowledge feelings without jumping ahead too quickly to try to do something: to use technical expertise to make things feel better without first having tried to really understand.

On the other hand, there is a risk that having needs for dependency met in this phase of treatment (both for the patient and perhaps indirectly for the practitioner) may mean that it is difficult to move on to the next phases of challenge and return to mutuality. There will come a time at which a change of emphasis is needed and this requires sensitivity and careful judgement about the patient's capacity for change and readiness to take more responsibility for his own well-being.

The practitioner also has a duty to use whatever means are available to her to develop an understanding of herself and, in particular, her own reactions to illness and dependency. This is important for several reasons: first, so that the practitioner can separate out her own feelings from those of her patient; second, so that she can use her own knowledge of herself as a guide to what the patient may be feeling; third, to make it less likely that she blocks off discomfort and distress; fourth, so that she is able to hold in awareness the fact that it could be herself in the patient's position. The practitioner's need to take care of herself will be considered further in Chapter 9.

Phase 4   Challenge

In this phase, the expert technical skills of the practitioner are brought into play in order either to challenge destructive or unhelpful beliefs or to challenge the symptoms of the disease or illness. Here the practitioner needs to be more authoritative and directive, but still within the context of a respectful, trusting and caring relationship. This is the phase of treatment where there is the greatest need for the practitioner to use her expert power.

Schaap et al (1993), in discussing cognitive therapy (a form of psychotherapy which challenges dysfunctional thoughts), noted that during the phase of treatment in which the techniques of change are used, clear directives are expected by patients and are experienced as helpful. The authors pointed out that while advice early in treatment is unhelpful, later it becomes inevitable and necessary. They also noted that there is a decrease in empathic statements later in treatment and that, although reflection of feelings may tend to generate trust at the beginning of treatment, getting stuck at this level may prevent constructive change. Insofar as illness consists of personal understandings as well as disease factors, change may require an alteration in the patient's conceptualization of and attitude towards the illness, including his own part in dealing with it. Thus, treatment includes helping the patient to reach a new, more constructive conceptualization of his illness.

A study of the effects of general practitioners' consulting styles on patients' satisfaction with treatment (Savage & Armstrong 1990) found that patients who received a directing style (assertive, authoritative statements from the doctor), as compared to a more sharing, discursive style, were more likely to feel that they had received an excellent explanation, that the GP had a complete understanding of their problem and, 1 week later, felt that they had been greatly helped. However, this benefit disappeared for patients who were judged to have chronic illnesses. The authors speculated that there may be two broad types of illness for which different consultation styles are more appropriate. Simple physical illness that responds to traditional biomedical approaches of diagnosis and treatment would seem to benefit from a more directing style. For chronic illnesses and those which have a large psychosocial component, this benefit disappears and perhaps a more sharing style may be more suitable.

Studies in orthodox medicine have raised the concern that many patients do not understand the advice given by their doctors and that between one-third and a half of all patients do not follow the advice of their doctors. There is some evidence that improved and clearer information giving reduces distress and speeds up recovery (Ley 1988). This involves giving the most important information first, repeating information, using shorter sentences and a simpler vocabulary, explicitly categorizing information and asking the patient to repeat information given. These are all examples of the practitioner behaving in an appropriately authoritative manner.

Phase 5   Return to mutuality

Within the model, there is a return to mutuality towards the end of treatment, with a more equal and balanced therapeutic relationship. This phase may be reached temporarily at the end of each treatment session during a course of treatment or, more permanently, when a course of treatment is ending.

Some practitioners will have a continuing therapeutic relationship with patients who remain 'on their books', perhaps for life, returning at intervals for help when needed. Others will have more limited and contained contracts, often with patients who come for specific treatment with specific problems. When the point has been reached when the patient and practitioner judge that the patient can continue to develop without the practitioner's help, then the therapeutic relationship can end, at least for the time being. Of course, for some patients with chronic and long-term conditions, the ending occurs only with the patient's death. In such a case, much of the treatment process will have been directed towards preparing for death itself.

Mutual respect

The power differences between patient and practitioner will have diminished as treatment comes towards the end. Ending can be helped by reviewing the progress which the patient has made and acknowledging his part in achieving change. If the treatment has been successful in empowering the patient, he will feel more in control of his health.

Creating positive expectations and recognition of limits

The patient's expectations of his future health should be considered towards the end of treatment. Clarifying the patient's responsibilities is important in order to facilitate the patient's own 'self-healing capacity': patients need to know what they can do in order to keep well. This phase of treatment therefore includes paying attention to self-help strategies needed to help with convalescence and to prevent or minimize the impact of future illness.

The recognition of limits requires the practitioner and patient to acknowledge again that some things may not be achievable. It may be that the patient will require treatment from the practitioner in the future: if so, the patient should be able to come back without feeling that he has failed. Indeed, some practitioners do suggest occasional follow-up treatments as a preventive measure. The practitioner might also help the patient to consider what resources are available to him for continued help and support in his family or social network. Finally, again, it may be a relief for the patient to be able to acknowledge the unchangeable aspects of his life and illness.

Shared understanding

At the end of treatment, it can be helpful for the practitioner to know what the patient has found useful, and less useful, in treatment. The patient can be encouraged by reminding himself of the changes which he has made.

In particular, the ending of treatment is another opportunity for the patient to try to make some sense of the illness in his life: he may again ask questions about the meaning of his illness and, indeed, about the deeper meanings of life and death. Reminiscence and attempts to make sense of life and death are particularly likely to happen at the end of treatment if the therapeutic relationship has been significant for a patient. The ending of treatment and of the therapeutic relationship may resonate with thoughts and feelings associated with previous losses in his life. The use of some sort of simple ritual to mark the ending may be beneficial in order to help the patient remind himself of what the illness, the treatment and the practitioner have meant to him and to help him to move on.

Ending treatment

A workshop with a group of complementary and orthodox health practitioners generated the following suggestions as ways of ensuring a constructive ending of treatment.

- Recognize that a good ending is based on having reached a shared understanding at the beginning of treatment.
- Use rituals and markers to make ending possible and meaningful.
- Manage ending in a way which enables the process of treatment to continue beyond the ending (mobilize self-healing).
- Help the patient to find sources of support in himself and others.
- Review what has happened in treatment and appropriately attribute success to the patient's efforts.
- Consider offering follow-up sessions as a safety net or as a preventive measure.
- Clarify whether, in what circumstances, and how, the patient could return for treatment.
- Consider ending sooner rather than later: some practitioners may maintain dependency inappropriately by continuing treatment for too long.
- Bear in mind that the ending may mirror previous losses.

- Convey a belief in the patient's capacity to take care of himself.
- Express love and concern in the farewell and acknowledge how both participants have valued the contact with one another.
- Acknowledge limitations: stop when the practitioner's and the patient's limits have been reached.

THE PROCESS OF TREATMENT: QUESTIONS FOR PRACTITIONERS

The following questions are designed for practitioners to check whether they are paying attention to the needs of patients throughout the process of treatment (following Bell (1994) who created a list of questions for clinical psychologists).

Mutuality

Mutual respect

- Are patients made to feel welcome and at ease when they arrive to see you, with a smile, handshake and somewhere comfortable to wait?
- Do you ask patients how they like to be addressed and tell them how they may address you?
- Do you explain the way you work, what the treatment will involve and what it will ask of your patient? Do you then discuss their views and give them the opportunity to consider before committing themselves to accepting treatment?
- Would your patients feel respected if they read the notes or letters you had written about them?
- What barriers may there be for some people in reaching your service (e.g. status, economic, class, race, gender, age, disability)?

Positive expectations and recognition of limits

- Do you feel confident and optimistic about the treatment methods you use? Do you keep up to date with new methods?
- Do you encourage patients in their own efforts to help themselves?

- Do you recognize your own professional and personal limits?
- Do you acknowledge the practical constraints operating on your patients' lives?
- Do you make positive use of ritual in your treatments?

Shared understanding

- Do you find out what other attempts your patients have made to deal with their illnesses?
- Do you ask patients about their own understandings of what their illness is, what has caused it, what may be stopping it from getting better and what needs to be done?
- Do you give patients the opportunity to explore the meaning and significance of their illness in their lives?
- Do you explain your formulation or diagnosis in words which the patient can understand?
- Do you reach a shared agreement with patients about the nature of the illness, what changes they would like to make and how you may help?

Trust

- Do you provide a treatment setting which meets patients' needs for access, modesty, comfort, confidentiality and dignity?
- Is there always someone else present nearby when you see patients, as a safeguard for you and your patients?
- Do you ask patients' permission before you discuss them with other professionals or when you write letters or make or respond to referrals?
- Do you understand the legal and moral codes relevant to your practice?
- Do patients know how they can make complaints if necessary?
- Do you continue to behave courteously and respectfully towards patients throughout treatment?
- Are you clear with patients, and do you give them choices, about such matters as how often they see you, when, where and whether they can contact you by letter or by telephone?
- Are you clear about the differences between friendship and therapeutic relationship?

- Are you understanding when patients are defensive (frightened) or reluctant to disclose information (wary)? Do you respect patients' rights not to disclose information when they choose not to?

Care

- Do you try to imagine things from your patients' point of view?
- Do you understand when problem behaviours (such as apparent unreasonableness, need for attention, lack of self-care) are a way of coping with unbearable or overwhelming feelings?
- Do you show patients that you can tolerate and accept their feelings?
- Are you thoughtful and careful about the use of touch?
- Do you remember how vulnerable patients might be?
- Do you use supervision and/or personal support to clarify your own feelings?
- Do you take account of your potential biases and preconceptions regarding gender, race, class, age and sexual orientation?
- Do you take care of yourself (e.g. by managing your time, paying enough attention to your family and friends, looking after your own spirit, mind and body, continuing to educate and refresh yourself)?

Challenge

- Do you explain the treatment techniques you use and their likely effects?
- Can you be clear, authoritative and decisive when necessary?
- Do you make sure that treatment makes sense to patients by explaining it in the context of their own understanding?
- Do you give advice in a way which the patient understands (using simple language, short sentences and asking them to repeat instructions)?
- Do you refrain from imposing your own ideas and values on patients?
- Do you help patients to change their attitudes and behaviours only when they want and are ready to do so?

Return to mutuality

- Do you return to a more equal relationship towards the end of treatment?
- When and if you reveal information about yourself, do you do so only to show that you are human and fallible too, not to show that you know best, nor that you know exactly what it is like to be the patient, nor to require the patient to take care of you?
- Do you give patients credit for the changes they have made?
- Do you explore with patients what might make the illness or difficulties return, so that they can consider the parts played by themselves and their environment in preventing recurrence?
- Are you aware of all the local resources which may be relevant to your patients' needs? Do you pass on to patients knowledge about relevant literature, self-help groups, sources of advice on financial matters, other treatment possibilities, other sources of knowledge and help?
- Do you involve patients in evaluating the service that you offer? Do you work towards improvements by incorporating the information and feedback provided by people who use, or reject, your services?

REFERENCES

Bandura A 1977 Self-efficacy: towards a unifying theory of behavior change. Psychological Review 84(2): 191–215
Bell I, 1994 Twenty questions: some pointers for good practice. Clinical Psychology Forum 66:29
Bennet G 1987 The wound and the doctor. Secker and Warburg, London
Berger P, Luckman T 1966 The social construction of reality. Penguin, Harmondsworth
Bowlby J 1969 Attachment and loss, vol 1. Attachment. Hogarth Press, London
Carroll D, Bennett P, Davey Smith G 1993 Socio-economic health inequalities: their origins and implications. Psychology and Health 8:295–316
Coward R 1989 The whole truth: the myth of alternative health. Faber and Faber, London
Frank J D 1973 Persuasion and healing, 2nd edn. Johns Hopkins University Press, Baltimore
Howe D 1993 On being a client. Sage, London
Kakar S 1982 Shamans, mystics and doctors: a psychological enquiry into India and its healing traditions. Knopf, New York
Kleinman A 1988 The illness narratives. Basic Books, New York

Ley P 1988 Communicating with patients: improving communication, satisfaction and compliance. Croom Helm, London

Mead G H 1934 Mind, self and society. University of Chicago Press, Chicago

Mitchell A 1995 The therapeutic relationship in health care: towards a model of the process of treatment. Journal of Interprofessional Care 9:15–20

Needleman J 1985 The way of the physician. Penguin, Harmondsworth

Richards M P M 1974 The integration of a child into a social world. Cambridge University Press, Cambridge

Richards M P M, Light P (eds) 1986 Children of social worlds: development in a social context. Polity Press, Cambridge

Richardson P 1989 Placebos: their effectiveness and modes of action. In: Broome A K (ed) Health psychology: processes and applications. Chapman and Hall, London

Roose-Evans J 1994 Passages of the soul: ritual today. Element Books, Shaftesbury

Savage R, Armstrong D 1990 Effect of general practitioners' consulting style on patients' satisfaction: a controlled study. British Medical Journal 301:968–970

Schaap C, Bennun I, Schindlet L, Hoogduin K 1993 The therapeutic relationship in behavioural psychotherapy. Wiley, Chichester

Skelton J A, Groyle R T 1991 Mental representation, health and illness: an introduction. In: Skelton J A, Groyle R T (eds) Mental representation in health and illness. Springer-Verlag, New York, ch 1

Skynner R 1986 What is effective in group psychotherapy? Group Analysis 19:5–24

Smail D 1994 Community psychology and politics. Journal of Community and Applied Social Psychology 42:3–10

Sperry R W, Gazzaniga M S, Bogen J E 1969 Inter-hemisphere relationships: the neocortical commissures: syndromes of hemisphere disconnection. In: Vinken P J, Bruyn G W (eds) Handbook of clinical neurology, vol 4. Disorders of speech, perception and symbolic behaviour. North Holland, Amsterdam, pp 273–290

Townsend P, Davidson N 1982 The Black report. Penguin, Harmondsworth

Tuckett D, Boulton M, Olson C, Williams A 1985 Meetings between experts. Tavistock Publications, London

Watts G 1992 Pleasing the patient. Faber and Faber, London

Wilkinson R G 1996 Unhealthy societies: the afflictions of inequality. Routledge, London

9

The health of the practitioner

There seems to be a paradox in our approach to thinking about the health of the practitioner. On one hand is the hope for the healer to seem invulnerable and beyond the reach of trouble and disorder, while on the other hand is the wish that the healer could understand, from her own personal experience, what suffering really feels like.

Practitioners and patients alike may collude in the fantasy that if the physician can symbolize perfect health, then somehow perfect health can be attainable and death can be warded off. In their book *When doctors get sick*, Mendell & Spiro (1987) suggested that the role of healer requires the physician to seem immune from disease. Practitioners themselves may experience pressure to seem inviolable, untouched by illness. Indeed, Bennet (1987) and Krakowski (1982) have argued that part of the motivation to become a doctor is to avoid or master the fear of death. Bennet described how doctors fear and avoid indications of mortality in themselves, their families and their colleagues. We do not yet know to what extent this holds true for complementary practitioners. We know of no research which has explored this area. The suggestion is that playing the role of healer can provide a means of denying one's own human vulnerability. Such a denial may, to some extent at least, prove effective in branches of medicine where cure is the norm; it is likely to break down in the face of chronic and life-threatening illness where the permanence and inevitability of suffering and death cannot be avoided.

Here the other side of the paradox comes to the fore: patients wish that the healers could *really* know what it is like to be suffering, through being open to the possibility of suffering themselves. This is one of the most powerful messages which can be taken from work with people with long-term health needs: patients wish practitioners would understand that they, too, could be in need of care, so that the barriers between 'them' and 'us' may be broken down and practitioners would be truly open to understanding things from the patients' point of view. 'If only they could realize, at a deep level, that any of them could become any one of us' (mother of daughter with multiple disabilities, personal communication to A Mitchell, 1994).

THE IDEA OF THE WOUNDED HEALER

The paradox may be resolved in the ancient mythical idea of the wounded healer, summed up in the aphorism attributed to Carl Jung: 'In the end, only the wounded physician heals'. Bennet (1987), psychiatrist and surgeon, in his book *The wound and the doctor*, returned to popular consciousness the idea contained in ancient Greek mythology that the capacities to harm and to heal, and to be harmed and to be healed, can co-exist within one person. This idea is exemplified in the mythical figure of Chiron, the centaur, who combined the wisdom of man with the instinctive power of the horse and taught the healing arts to Asclepius, son of Apollo, who went on to become one of the great healers featured in the Hippocratic oath. Chiron himself had been wounded by the poisoned arrow of Heracles; his wound never healed in his immortal state and he eventually traded immortality for mortality to bring his suffering to an end. As well as embodying deep knowledge of healing, Chiron was also expert in the arts of war and taught Achilles to become a successful and skilful warrior.

The story of Chiron, and those of other Greek figures including Hygeia and Panacea, are resonant with the notion of a healer being someone who has the power to harm and to heal and yet also has weakness and vulnerability symbolized by the possession of a wound. The shamanistic tradition, too, accepts and sometimes requires the healer to be someone who has been troubled in some way and who has mastered trauma or disease in himself. In shamanism, chosen healers may have a physical impairment or affliction or may have experienced some sort of emotional or spiritual breakdown from which they have emerged strengthened. This mystical quality of the power of the healer's wounds is a central theme in Christian teaching, too, exemplified in the person of Jesus as a healer who carried a wound and of whom we are told by Peter, 'by his wounds you are healed.' Bennet, in an earlier paper, expounded:

The essential feature is not merely that the healer has endured affliction but has gone on to assimilate the experience of it, either to be cured or to learn to live with the wound as a creative part of the healer's being. (Bennet 1984: 129)

Why might the wounded healer have the power to heal?

What is it about someone who, as a healer, has herself been wounded which gives her a particular power to heal? There are three possibilities to consider: the wounded healer may be able to activate the patient's own inner powers of recuperation; the wounded healer may be able to inspire the patient through her own example; the wounded healer may be able to understand the patient's experience.

The wounded healer may be able to activate the patient's own inner powers of recuperation

This suggestion is based on the implications of the healer–patient archetype, introduced in Chapter 7. The underlying concept is inherent in most prescientific philosophical systems: everything exists only in relation to its opposite. This implies the relationship between polarities: there can be no light without dark, no female without male, no up without down, no patient without healer. Moreover, inherent in the existence of one pole or extreme is the potential for the existence of the other pole. Thus, instead of thinking that any one person is *either* only-a-healer *or* only-a-patient, we can think of the inner healer *in* the patient and of the inner patient *in* the healer. Both Bennet (1987) and Guggenbühl-Craig (1971) indicated that being a healer and being healed are not mutually exclusive. To the extent that the healer can convey her awareness of her potential for being a patient (her symbolic wound), then the patient may be able to activate his own intrinsic capacity for being a healer and thus contribute to his own self-healing.

Given the powerful expectations about practitioners' health, it would hardly be surprising if practitioners were, at best, ambivalent about their own vulnerability. Walsh et al (1991) found that, for clinical psychologists, the possibility of *themselves* becoming clients in need of therapy was linked with notions such as being less coping, less able, less powerful, lost, defeated, a burden or a source of strain. Does this mean that clinical psychologists view their patients in these negative terms? And what efforts may be put into shoring up the professional's own sense of personal health to ward off feelings of vulnerability? The implication here is that it may be more healthy, for all concerned, to acknowledge that practitioners are as vulnerable to the vicissitudes of life as the next person. Recognizing this may relieve practitioners from the impossible burden of seeming the all-powerful, all-knowing, perfect healers. At the same time, such acknowledgement may free patients to find or use their own personal power, knowledge and strength which otherwise would be owned and carried only by the apparently omnipotent practitioner. This would then facilitate the patient's more active participation in the treatment and in the healing process. Certainly, this is the aim in most complementary treatment.

Conveying to patients the possibility of the practitioner's vulnerability requires tact, delicacy and sensitivity to the requirements of the particular situation. It can never be justified to burden patients with self-revelations of distress, neediness or, indeed, of success in coping. It would be only too easy for patients to slip to the other extreme and take on a sense of responsibility for the practitioner's well-being. It is probable that during the active phases of personal distress and suffering, practitioners are less likely to have the capacity to be helpful to patients. Wounds need to be healed, or at least to be healing, before the experiences they bring can be drawn on as a resource: they should be scars rather than open wounds. When the practitioner is actively ill or openly distressed, the responsible course of action is to take time off from seeing patients.

The practitioner's acknowledgement of personal vulnerability should usually be implicit rather than explicit. She would then come across in the consultation as an approachable, real person who is familiar and comfortable with physical and emotional suffering. Such a practitioner would be able to witness, contain and bear the patient's pain and would work together with the patient to find active ways of managing and coping, rather than, on the one hand, brusquely pushing away any emotional expression or, on the other, becoming overwhelmed and hopeless in the face of distress.

The wounded healer may be able to inspire the patient through her own example

The suggestion here is that if the practitioner knows, through direct personal experience, that affliction can be overcome or lived with, then she can offer hope and inspiration to the patient. This hope can be conveyed to the patient either directly or indirectly.

Oliver Sacks, in his account of his own experience as a patient when he lost the use of his leg, referred to in Chapter 3, gave an excellent example of a doctor acting as a role model who exemplified that it is possible to overcome affliction. Sacks had just had his broken leg set temporarily in a cast, and the young surgeon treating him showed him his own scars from broken thighs in skiing accidents:

Of all the doctors I had ever seen, or was later to see, the image of this young Norwegian surgeon remains most vividly and affectionately in my mind, because in *his own person* he stood for health, valour, humour – and a most wonderful, active empathy for patients. He didn't talk like a textbook. He scarcely talked at all – he acted. He leapt and danced and showed me his wounds, showing me at the same time his perfect recovery. His visit made me feel immeasurably better. (Sacks 1991: 26)

The message to the patient here is clear and unambiguous: *if it is possible for me to do it, then it is possible for you to do it too.* In this case, the practitioner acts as a sort of coping role model, someone who sets an example which the patient can follow. The practitioner need not necessarily display her (literal or metaphorical) wounds directly to the patient. It may be that her knowledge, based on direct personal experience that suffering can be survived and overcome will give her a sense of real authority. This authority may inspire the patient's trust and belief in her. At the same time, this authority can give her a confidence which may inspire the patient to begin to take whatever action is needed for him to cope with his illness.

The wounded healer may be able to understand the patient's experience

The wounded healer really knows what it is like to suffer and so may be better able to be actively empathic and to understand what it is that patients may want and need within the therapeutic relationship. Many first-person accounts of doctors' and other practitioners' personal experiences of illness convey the message that it was not until they had been ill themselves that they knew properly how to treat patients. Thus, for example, in their book on mental health workers' experiences of depression, Rippere & Williams (1985) found that the single most frequent comment made by practitioners who had been depressed, when asked what lessons they had learnt from their experience, was that it gave more understanding of, and empathy with, depressed patients.

The specifics of the lessons reflected the individual experiences. They included recognizing the importance of relating to patients as whole and potentially viable people, of encouraging them rather than trying to destroy their defences in the name of some abstract therapeutic ideology, of refraining from judging, and of listening, trying to respond to patients' needs, and trying to provide the kind of help they want. (Rippere & Williams 1985: 183–184)

For those practitioners who have not themselves been directly exposed to the same sorts of distress or suffering that their patients experience, reading first-hand accounts is an excellent way of gaining an insight into people's subjective experience. This is the sort of essential knowledge which is rarely included in academic textbooks or in professional training.

WHAT IS KNOWN ABOUT ILLNESS IN PRACTITIONERS?

Much has been written about the vulnerability of health care workers to stress and burnout (British Medical Association 1992, Burnard 1991, Edelwich & Brodsky 1980, Maslach 1981, Paine 1982, Pines & Aronson 1988). Let us begin this section by examining what is known about illness experienced by health care workers. At the outset, we should state that we know of no published work which looks at the health and illness of complementary practitioners in particular. Clearly there is scope for investigation here. Most that is written on this subject is based on studies of medical doctors and, to a lesser extent, nurses. The situation for complementary practitioners may be quite different.

In comparison with other professional groups, doctors have relatively good physical health but relatively poor psychological health and nurses have relatively poor physical and psychological health (Sutherland & Cooper 1990). Doctors are at increased risk of alcohol and drug abuse (Bennet 1987). They also have a high risk of dying from causes considered to be related to stress: suicide, cirrhosis of the liver and poisoning accidents. Overall, reports suggest that male doctors are about twice as likely to commit suicide than males from other professional groups and female doctors are at an even greater risk. Krakowski (1982) reported that female doctors' suicide risk is four times that of other professional women. Nurses, too, have an increased risk of suicide relative to other professional women, have high rates of psychiatric outpatient referrals and high rates of absenteeism and work drop-out.

These published findings are the tip of the iceberg, underlying which may be a great deal of distress; hence the recent concern to look in more detail at the nature of stress at work and at 'burnout'.

WHAT ARE STRESS AND BURNOUT?

In simple terms, a person becomes overstressed when demands exceed perceived resources. The notions of 'demands' and 'resources' alert us to the necessity, when considering the nature and impact of stress, to look both at the individual person who is experiencing the stress *and* at the social system within which she is operating, which may or may not provide her with the coping resources she needs and which may or may not in itself be a source of demands.

A reasonable amount of stress is inevitable and, indeed, positive in activating our bodies, minds and spirits. It awakens our energy in readiness for action. However, more stress than can be managed may translate into physical, mental, emotional and behavioural symptoms. Some of the more common symptoms of stress in practitioners are listed in Table 1; perhaps other warning signals of excess stress could be added.

It is suggested that if someone is constantly exposed to a situation in which demands exceed resources, her energies will

Table 1 Symptoms of excess stress

Physical
1. Headaches and other bodily pains
2. Diarrhoea, indigestion, constipation
3. Sleep disturbance
4. Overtiredness
5. Appetite loss

Mental
1. A reduced ability to concentrate
2. Increased forgetfulness
3. Constant worry
4. Seeing oneself as a victim
5. Expectation of blame

Behavioural
1. Behaving as a carer but not feeling caring
2. Avoiding clients, colleagues, situations
3. Turning to drink, overeating, oversmoking
4. Frequent lateness
5. Loss of a sense of humour

Emotional
1. Sudden swings in feelings
2. Bouts of crying
3. Floating anxiety
4. Resenting patients
5. Low mood

(adapted from Hawkins & Shohet 1989)

gradually deplete, culminating in the state of emotional and physical apathy and exhaustion known as 'burnout' (Maslach & Jackson 1981). It is as if some sort of balance or equation is in operation: the person can continue working effectively and with satisfaction if the physical and emotional energy put into work is balanced with some sort of return, regulated by the person's own recuperative capacity. However, if her resources are continually depleted, eventually she will have nothing left to give.

The term 'burnout' was introduced by Freudenberger & Richelson (1974) to describe the emotional and physical exhaustion experienced by front-line community workers dealing with the intractable problems and distress of people with mental health difficulties. An early definition of burnout encompassed three areas.

1. *Emotional exhaustion*: being overextended and drained by others

2. *Depersonalization*: a callous response to the recipients of
   services
3. *Reduced personal accomplishment*: a decline in feelings of
   competence and successful achievement.
   (Maslach & Jackson 1981)

What leads to burnout and what can be done to prevent it?

The seeds of potential burnout, which may be targets for possible
efforts at prevention, can be identified at three levels.

1. *The individual practitioner*: are there any personal
   characteristics which may make someone vulnerable or
   resistant to burnout?
2. *The practitioner–patient relationship*: is there anything
   distinctive about the therapeutic relationship which may be
   linked with burnout?
3. *The working environment*: what are the factors in the social or
   organizational setting which may reduce or increase the risk
   of burnout?

The individual practitioner

Hawkins & Shohet (1989) suggested that, insofar as the potential
for burnout resides in the personal characteristics of the practitioner, then the best time to attend to burnout is before it
happens.

This involves looking at your shadow motivation for being in the
helping professions . . . monitoring your own stress symptoms and
managing a healthy support system . . . and ensuring that you have a
meaningful, enjoyable and physically active life outside the role of being
a helper. (Hawkins & Shohet 1989: 20)

The suggestion here is that part of the motivation for becoming a
practitioner lies outside our conscious awareness and that some
unconscious needs may drive us to work beyond the bounds of
reasonableness and in the end to the detriment, rather than to
the benefit, of patients as well as ourselves.

There are probably as many different and complex motivations
underlying people's choice of career as there are people making
the choices. In some ways there may be particular motivational

issues for complementary practitioners as compared with orthodox practitioners, since a greater proportion move into their careers as helpers later in life rather than, as for most doctors and nurses, in their young adulthood. Much of what is thought about the motivation underlying the choice of a career as a helper is drawn from the study of doctors, so it is important to be cautious about drawing too many conclusions. We really need to know more about the backgrounds, experiences and motivations of complementary practitioners.

Despite these caveats, some general themes can be drawn from what has been written about practitioners' motives. Such motives seem to range from the fully conscious, easily accessible and straightforwardly altruistic desire to offer ourselves and our skills in the service of others, to have work which is stimulating, challenging and meaningful and to work in professions which may value our particular combination of skills and abilities through to wanting a career which offers some degree of status, prestige and financial security and less conscious motivations deriving from our own early experiences of care and caring. Hawkins & Shohet (1989) agree with other writers (including Bennet 1987, Guggenbühl-Craig 1971, Hillman 1979) that a willingness to examine our own deeper motives, 'good' or 'bad', pure or complex, is a prerequisite for being an effective helper.

Following Jung, and in the tradition of Freudian psychodynamic theory which considers some aspects of motivation to be outside conscious awareness, we can consider the 'shadow side' of choosing to become a helper, which may include offering help to others as a way of doing one, some or all of the following.

- Warding off thoughts of our own mortality or our own craziness
- Continuing to be sensitive to others' needs because this was what we had to do in our own early life
- Looking for ways to allow ourselves and others to believe we are special so as to shore up our own shaky self-esteem
- Gaining power and control over others
- Finding a way of being intimate without having to reveal all of ourselves
- Giving to others as a way of gaining reparation for the love and care we wish we had received in childhood

- Indulging our prurient fascination with the lives and troubles of others
- Feeling good in ourselves in contrast to others' suffering.

The list could go on; the point is that our motives may not all be 'nice' and also that we inevitably express our own needs to some extent in our choice of work. It is considered that it is not the needs in themselves which are dangerous, but rather their denial. Needs which are denied may become imperatives, so that we act out of compulsion rather than choice. Being aware of our own shadow, it is hoped, will make us more open to the needs of the patient and less likely to be offering help which is driven by ourselves rather than by the needs of particular patients with whom we are faced. We all have complicated and legitimate needs and desires to help and be helped; the problem for us comes when these are met *only* in our work as therapists, not also in our wider life. Personal awareness through thoughtful reflection can help us to be sensitive to the times when our own motivation is intruding into our service of patients' needs.

Hawkins & Shohet (1989) made the important point that the idea of being a helper, as opposed to simply a vehicle or channel for help, is a tricky one. It makes us addicted to praise, fearful of blame and keeps us on the seesaw between impotence and omnipotence which distracts from the patient's potential for power. The concept of 'non-attachment' may be attractive to complementary practitioners since it implies that it is really the patient who does the healing, rather than the practitioner.

Non-attachment does not mean not caring. On the contrary it may be the nearest we can get to real caring as we do not have to live through our clients, dependent on their successes for our self-esteem. (Hawkins & Shohet 1989: 9)

The practitioner–patient relationship

The corollary of the argument outlined above is that correcting the imbalance between giving and receiving help may be in the interests of both practitioner and patient; less compulsive giving on the part of the practitioner frees the patient to use his own inner strength. A realignment of the healer–patient archetype can open up the possibility for the therapeutic relationship to be healing for the practitioner as well as for the patient. The suggestion here is that practitioners who are able to have more equal and mutually balanced relationships with their patients may be less prone to depletion of their resources (and hence less likely to become burnt out) and are able to learn and develop through their practice.

The working environment

Often the features of work stress that may result in burnout are more to do with the organization and power structures of jobs than with the central tasks of the occupation. People who care for individuals with terminal illness may, from a layman's perspective, quite obviously be in stressful jobs. Research indicates that it is not patient distress and death which are the central features of burnout; it is the management of the organizations and the minutiae of day-to-day administrative activities which are the subject of complaint and are identified as the sources of stress and burnout (Sutherland & Cooper 1990). Lack of autonomy, non-involvement in decision making, excessive paper work, unpredictable changes in routine, unclear rules and regulations and excessive demands from work supervisors are the straws that break the backs of people coping heroically with emotionally demanding and challenging jobs. When people work in comparative isolation, with few opportunities for communication about their difficulties, no support provided in their work and no sense of their tasks being valued within the organization, then vulnerability to stress and burnout increases.

To the extent that complementary practitioners do work autonomously, they may be protected from some of the negative pressures of organizational settings, such as are inherent within the NHS, but equally their independence may isolate them from sources of support which could help them to cope with the stresses they do feel.

It is the case that many complementary practitioners do not have access to support and supervision in their working lives. In a survey of personal support for complementary practitioners, only one-third had any professional supervision and more than half of those without supervision wanted some way of finding it (Mitchell, unpublished work, 1995). Only half of the practitioners had any form at all of personal support at work and most people wanted more support than was currently available to them.

The answers to the question 'What stops you from having supervision or support?' revealed practical and logistic reasons. There were no formal mechanisms for support or supervision, and practitioners would have had to pay for any time lost from clinical contact. Moreover, many practitioners valued their independence and were a little suspicious that support systems in themselves may prove to be emotionally, as well as practically and economically, costly. There was also some personal resistance to receiving support, hinted at in some replies in which practitioners mentioned inhibitions, through low self-esteem and loss of pride at admitting failure.

Clinical work was seen as having personal benefits and costs. Costs included demands on one's own time, with consequent negative effects on family life. People mentioned the emotionally tiring or draining effect of clinical work, along with physical tiredness. Some commented on having that 'past caring feeling', having 'had enough of people by the end of the day' and finding it 'hard to give at home after giving all day'. Others emphasized the personal benefits of clinical work, such as fulfilment and satisfaction when the work goes well, appreciating the flexibility of the working hours and feeling that the rewards outweighed the costs.

Practitioners were aware of a potential imbalance in terms of giving out energy to patients while gradually becoming personally drained, so that practitioners' families sometimes suffered. Practitioners were clear that it is important, though not always easy, to maintain and restore one's own resources.

Ways of looking after themselves which were most frequently mentioned were: keeping up to date with new knowledge, protecting family time, physical self-help (care over eating, sleeping, relaxation and exercise), using therapies themselves and, less frequently, keeping up regular contact with colleagues. One person succinctly summed up self-care as 'Eat well, sleep well, read well, relax well and love life' – a formula which we would all do well to follow.

BARRIERS TO SELF-CARE

It is a curious irony that we who are in the helping professions sometimes do not apply what we know about self-care to our own lives. Again, it is as if we may feel one or all of the following.

- It can't happen to me: I am invulnerable – so I don't need to look after myself.
- I don't deserve to be cared for in the same ways as others.
- I can't get sick because others depend on me.
- My job is to look after others, not to look after myself.
- Taking holidays or time off is a major tribulation because the demands of work pile up.

If we overcome the barriers and manage to look after ourselves well, we can enhance our own capacity to look after others, which is what we aspire consciously to do. The first task, then, in taking care of our own health is to recognize that we have a responsibility to do so, since we can only be in a position to give when our own needs have, at least to some extent, been acknowledged and satisfied.

PRACTITIONERS' HEALTH: IMPLICATIONS FOR PRACTICE

Levels of self-care
• Individual level • Relationship level • Social context.

As individuals

Explore motivation before becoming a healer

Acknowledge and celebrate your straightforwardly altruistic motives and allow yourself to enjoy and appreciate your capacity to give to others. Attempt to identify your more hidden motivations for becoming a healer to help you to recognize when you may be being driven by your own needs rather than by the demands of the situation.

Find ways to maintain interest, enthusiasm and knowledge

- Remain alert to new ideas in practice and in the literature.
- Combat the isolation of your work by attending conferences,

workshops, courses and lectures and discussing your practice with other people.

- Allow your career to oscillate through periods of intense absorption in work (for instance during training) balanced by shifts when other aspects of life are to the fore.
- Consider forming a regular group to share your new knowledge and benefit from the experiences of others. Interest and enthusiasm are maintained by sharing with others and can quickly wane if there is very little feedback on what you are doing.
- Ensure that you hear and accept the praise from patients who have benefited from your work.
- Share some of your professional concerns with trusted colleagues in the hope of gaining reassurance about your own skills.

Exercise to explore personal motivation

This exercise to reflect on your own motivation can be done on your own or with the help of a friend or colleague to talk you through it.

Take some time to relax (in whatever way you find easiest) and allow yourself to return in your memory to some significant times through your development. For each point, do what you can to recall yourself and your situation at that time (place, sights, smells, textures, sizes, sounds, familiar people, objects, positions). Consider reflecting on the following periods.

- Some time before starting school
- Early childhood – maybe while at primary school
- Growing up – perhaps around the time of puberty
- Leaving home
- Young adulthood – setting up your own home
- Beginning professional training
- Following birth of children (if you have them)
- Around the death of a significant person.

At each point, recall:

- Who was around to look after you at that time?
- What did they do to look after you?
- Who did you look after at that time?
- What did you do to look after them?

Finally, how do these recollections connect with your life now?

This exercise can be profound and unsettling. Be careful to give yourself plenty of time for reflection afterwards and be prepared for further memories and reflections to return later. It can be a useful source of ideas and thoughts about why you want to offer help to others now.

Look after body, mind and spirit

It goes without saying that we all need to have a balanced life, with enough sleep, leisure, exercise, rest, creative activity, meaningful relationships and fun to balance the potentially draining quality of work. People who enjoy their jobs and survive well are those who:

- pace their work appropriately
- gain stimulation and enjoyment from the tasks they undertake
- move from work to home or leisure with a clear sense of leaving work behind
- set limits and have priorities other than work (this can lead to more effective and fruitful practice, because you are fresher and have a clearer perspective)
- take physical exercise which is aerobic (cardiovascular exercise has been shown to improve mood and lead to greater psychological health)
- practise spiritual exercises, especially meditation, which help people to focus more clearly and to gain meaning and harmonious balance in their lives.

Within the relationship between practitioner and patient

Recognize the interdependence of the patient and practitioner

Just as the practitioner has to be conscious of the responsibility and power that is held and be sensitive about not abusing her position, so patients also need to know the rules of the game. Practitioners can be drained by the demands of patients and need to establish clear boundaries and agreed expectations of patient behaviour and demands. Patients need to know what practitioners cannot do, as well as what they can do. This can be done by:

- offering clear information, possibly in leaflets that patients can take home
- explaining your treatment aims, methods and limitations
- encouraging patients to ask questions about your practice
- creating a structure so that the patient knows when you are, and are not, available.

Identify what the patient really wants

Understanding the patient's needs and his reasons for coming to the consultation provides a framework for a more rewarding interaction. It is certainly the case that sometimes patients may want explanation or practical advice, reassurance or a listening ear, rather than the solution to very difficult or intractable problems. Being realistic about what can be achieved can be a relief for the practitioner as well as for the patient and saves both from the disappointment of failing to achieve unrealistically high expectations.

Maintain appropriate boundaries

It is helpful for both patient and practitioner to keep to set starting and finishing times for appointments. It is especially important with distressed or vulnerable patients to whom it is tempting to give more time. If the practitioner takes responsibility for the time keeping, then the patient can feel safe to use the time productively. Both patient and practitioner can benefit from good management of time. Useful ways of ending a session are to forewarn the patient that there are only a few minutes left or to have a routine question to use before the end, such as, 'Is there anything more to discuss before we end?'.

Personal life needs to be protected and this can be a difficulty when the practitioner works from home. Having a business telephone line which is only answered at certain times and has an answerphone message indicating when you may be available can be extremely useful. You can also explain that messages may be intercepted at certain specified times. Time should be allocated during the normal working day to allow for this activity.

In the broader social context

Recognize constraints and limitations

The role of the practitioner needs to be clarified and untangled from notions about being perfectly strong, healthy, in control and omnipotent. Practitioners are not infallible and cannot be expected to deal with everything. Many of the sources of distress lie in social and environmental factors which are outside the scope of any one individual to change. You therefore do not need to feel guilty about being stressed in response to events which are outside your control.

Practitioners are just as prone to illness, stress, distress and self-doubt as anyone else and need to recognize that they cannot cure all their own ills. Having your own doctor or alternative practitioner to whom you can take your illness or stress recognizes that part of appropriate treatment is an alternative viewpoint on the trouble and a perspective of new ideas.

Remember that there are limits to what can be achieved with individual patients. Consider complementing your therapeutic endeavours with social or political activity, either locally or in a broader context, or find ways of being effective in the world other than through offering treatment (e.g. through sport, teaching, influencing professional organizations).

Identifying sources of personal and social support

Support needs to come from a variety of sources. Networking, having regular meetings for supervision, sharing ideas and developing mutual trust with others can be very important sources of support. It is sometimes as much the act of sharing as the resultant support and advice which is helpful. The interplay of ideas can suggest new avenues to explore and give hope of resolution or else confirm that the problem is truly outside the control of the individual.

POSITIVE BENEFITS OF BEING A PRACTITIONER

Having considered the issues which need addressing to prevent stress and burnout, we must also celebrate the positive side of giving health care to others. The rewards of the work are self-evident: the task is exciting, challenging and creative. Tackling a patient's health concerns involves the thrill of problem solving, stretching the practitioner's mind and often results in further learning from the patient. The underlying motivations for the work exist because, for many of us, there is an intrinsic, straight-forward pleasure in being able to relate to and help another person. Personal satisfaction comes from the rewards of seeing suffering reduced and from the gratitude expressed by the patient. At a different level, there is fulfilment from recognizing the altruistic value of helping an individual to be more capable of continuing in his societal role. Healing is thus beneficial not just for the patient and practitioner, but also for society in demonstrating our interdependence as citizens and our social and survival needs to help each other towards well-being.

Within the notion of the wounded healer, the one who has overcome her suffering, is the benefit of the personal development that ensues from the recovery. We can learn a great deal from being unwell, enriching us for future work. Grounding theory and knowledge in personal experience adds a dimension of meaning which can lead to greater empathy, understanding and compassion. Equally, we can learn a great deal from how our patients tackle distress. The learning to be gained from successive encounters with patients provides satisfying personal and professional development when the practitioner is open to incorporating new ideas and knowledge into her framework of understanding. Personal development also comes from experiencing with patients their suffering and growing through the humbling process of sharing in their pain.

In terms of preventing and dealing with stress, the practitioner is better equipped than most to recognize warning signs and symptoms of stress. Complementary health care approaches are often particularly suited to helping with stress, both in terms of keeping the body and mind healthy and directly tackling some of the results of stress. Recognition of the interplay between psyche and soma in the holistic approach, central to complementary therapies, can help the practitioner to become aware of stress at an early stage and to work effectively to overcome it. The balance between stimulating, challenging work and toil, which stresses the system, is a delicate one which needs careful and consistent monitoring. Through good attention to self-care, the complementary practitioner can achieve satisfying work and rich personal development.

REFERENCES

Bennet G 1984 The wounded healer in the twentieth century: re-evaluation of an ancient idea. British Journal of Holistic Medicine 1(2):127–130
Bennet G 1987 The wound and the doctor. Secker and Warburg, London
British Medical Association 1992 Stress and the medical profession. British Medical Association, London

Burnard P 1991 Coping with stress in the health professions: a practical guide. Chapman and Hall, London

Edelwich J, Brodsky A 1980 Burnout – stages of disillusionment in the helping professions. Human Sciences Press, New York

Freudenberger H, Richelson G 1974 Burnout: how to beat the high cost of success. Bantam Books, New York

Guggenbühl-Craig A 1971 Power in the helping professions. Spring, Dallas

Hawkins P, Shohet R 1989 Supervision in the helping professions. Open University Press, Buckingham

Hillman J 1979 In search: psychology and religion. Spring, Dallas

Krakowski A J 1982 Stress and the practice of medicine – the myth and the reality. Journal of Psychosomatic Research 26(1):91–98

Maslach C 1981 Burnout: the cost of caring. Prentice-Hall, Englewood Cliffs, New Jersey

Maslach C, Jackson S E 1981 The measurement of experienced burnout. Journal of Occupational Behaviour 2:99–113

Mendell H, Spiro H 1987 When doctors get sick. Plenum Press, New York

Paine W S (ed) 1982 Job stress and burnout: research, theory and intervention perspectives. Sage, Beverly Hills

Pines A, Aronson E 1988 Career burnout: causes and cures. Free Press, New York

Rippere V, Williams R 1985 Wounded healers: mental health workers' experiences of depression. Wiley, London

Sacks O 1991 A leg to stand on, revised edn. Picador, London

Sutherland V J, Cooper C L 1990 Understanding stress: a psychological perspective for health professionals. Chapman and Hall, London

Walsh S, Nichols K, Cormark M A 1991 Self-care and clinical psychologists — a threatening obligation? Clinical Psychology Forum 37: 5–7

10

Conclusion: centrality of the therapeutic relationship

This book began with the hope that it might help practitioners to reflect on how best to use themselves to promote the healing of their patients. We have looked at the therapeutic process through mutuality, trust, care, challenge and a return to mutuality. We have explored aspects of the therapeutic relationship: warmth, empathy, genuineness, authority, respect, collaborative communication, power and love.

It can sometimes seem as if there is a set of desired qualities, ownership of which may imbue the practitioner with some sort of special power. But to think in this way is to miss the point that it is the *relationship*, not the individual *person*, which can provide the framework for change. We have seen that the all-perfect healer is unlikely to be able to help patients to use their own healing energy. The healer needs to be a real person with her own characteristic weaknesses and strengths, vulnerabilities and powers. Any search for the nature of the healing self is illusory. The healer uses herself therapeutically simply by being herself and by being open and responsive to the needs of the other person; in so doing, she provides for the possibility of a real relationship in which the patient can heal. No-one can tell another person how to be herself. Being yourself cannot be done self-consciously or deliberately; it just happens, in the way that growth and development just happen, when the conditions are good enough to enable life to flourish.

This book is about how to create conditions good enough to facilitate growth, development and healing. Creating the right conditions, providing a framework, needs to be approached with concentration, thoughtfully and carefully, and in a way which allows for the personal style of the practitioner while respecting the individuality of the patient. Once the conditions are secure, the practitioner can put herself, with her knowledge, skills and techniques, at the patient's service. Yet, paradoxically, trying too hard to get it right may inhibit the therapeutic relationship. We hope that the ideas and suggestions in this book will encourage the reader to feel confident and at ease with her own approach to treatment. The conditions for healing rely as much on our shared understanding as on our clinical expertise. In this final chapter we want to return to some of the themes and issues recurring throughout the book in order to clarify why and how therapeutic relationships may heal.

HEALTH, ILLNESS AND HEALING

We began by differentiating health from the continuum of disease, illness and sickness. We have argued that a person may be more or less healthy, irrespective of whether or not he is ill. Someone may be faced with an acute or chronic illness, with a life-threatening disorder or with the certainty of death, yet it may be dealt with in a healthy way if it is used as an opportunity for the development of the person, the family or the wider social network. Equally, a person may be healthy, robust and resilient, yet be stricken with internal malfunctioning or external forces which may render him diseased or ill. Disease can be considered as a primary malfunctioning in biological or psychological processes, illness as the individual's experience of being 'out of order' and sickness as the social expression of disorder.

Health can be viewed from two perspectives: that of the individual who is striving to grow and develop and that provided by the environmental, social and cultural context which may facilitate or constrain the opportunities for individual development. We must acknowledge the dilemma of the practitioner who understands that the individual's power and capacity to maintain his own health is limited by the setting in which he lives. Individuals, either as patients or practitioners, do not have unlimited choice about, or control over, lifestyles and circumstances. Indeed, there is a risk that excessive attention to the promotion of 'healthy living' may lead to a preoccupation with health over other aspects of living, to undue interference with and moralizing judgement about people's ways of life and to increasing social sanction for those who are seen as 'failing' to remain healthy.

Thus, we recognize that too great a focus on the individual obscures the structural differences in society that affect health, by assuming that all individuals have an equal opportunity to live the kind of life that those who wish to promote health recommend. Yet individual practitioners, faced with individual patients, wish to empower patients to take an active stance in relation to their health, to encourage them to view themselves as other than passive victims of chance and to enable them to feel more in control. To do so requires a sensitive balance between acknowledging the limitations of circumstance and promoting realistic hope, optimism and confidence. An important aim of treatment is to help people to feel the best they can, irrespective of their circumstances.

COMPLEXITY AND FLOW

In Chapter 2 we defined health as development and suggested that part of the practitioner's task is to facilitate the development of the individual patient. A helpful perspective on the nature of this task is provided by the psychologist Csikszentmihalyi (1992) who has written about complexity and the growth of the self. Following Piaget, he suggested that development is a process through which the person becomes increasingly complex as a result of two broad psychological processes: differentiation and integration. Differentiation is a movement towards individuality, uniqueness, towards separating oneself from others. Integration is the opposite: a movement towards union, joining, towards connecting oneself with others. Complexity involves combining these opposing tendencies, leading to the integration of autonomous parts. A complex self is one who succeeds in becoming more his or her own self through connection with others. Development occurs through the increasing complexity of the individual within a social setting.

Interestingly, Csikszentmihalyi is able to cast new light on the notion of psychic energy, referred to by Needleman (1985) in Chapter 7. Csikszentmihalyi defined psychic energy as focused attention. He described the nature of what he has called 'flow experiences': those times when people typically feel strong, alert, in effortless control, unselfconscious and at the peak of their abilities. Such experiences, he argued, come about through a state of deep concentration in which consciousness is unusually well ordered: thoughts, intentions, feelings and all the senses become focused on the same goal. This is the state of focused attention, in which experience is in harmony. He argued that after a flow episode is over, 'One feels more "together" than before, not only internally but also with respect to the world in general' (Csikszentmihalyi 1992: 41). Such experiences are more likely to take place when the person feels safe and secure, when his or her attention is not distracted by competing demands.

There is a parallel to be drawn here with the nature of the healing act. First, as we described in Chapter 3, a healing act is one which pulls together the separate components of treatment (techniques, theory, practical action and the therapeutic relationship) into a complex whole. Second, we have noted the chaotic, disintegrating, disconnected nature of the experience of illness and have contrasted this with the experience of health in which people can take for granted their capacity just to get on with life. Cassell (1978) has described how the ill person feels separate from the world and loses any sense of personal power and control. Third, Needleman (1985) argued that healing involves re-invoking and channelling the person's 'will', his 'psychic energy' or his motivation, his desire to become well again. In Csikszentmihalyi's terms, this means establishing control over attention and focusing attention on becoming well. Most of us, as patients and practitioners, will recognize the quality of sustained attention which occurs when the concentration of the practitioner and patient together are focused on the task in hand.

This notion of flow, or focused attention, is important in consideration of the therapeutic relationship. It provides a way of ordering and understanding the practitioner's role in treatment. Csikszentmihalyi summarized the rules for facilitating flow experiences: setting clear goals which are commensurate with the person's abilities yet which are also challenging; becoming deeply immersed in the activity; focusing on immediate experience; paying close attention to what is happening. Attention refers not just to attending to the person but to what you are doing with the patient. This reminds us of the essential role of practised techniques and skills in treatment. It is important that we should not allow our awareness of the significance of the therapeutic relationship in treatment to lull us into thinking that we can thereby neglect the discipline or rigorous practice of technical skills or that we can be less than thorough in our understanding of the conceptual underpinning of our particular discipline. Rather, a working knowledge of the nature and effectiveness of the ideas and techniques of our disciplines will enhance our conviction and competence as practitioners and thereby form a safe framework for compassionate and productive therapeutic relationships.

If the practitioner follows Csikszentmihalyi's rules for her own practice, then she is likely to set the conditions in which the patient, too, is enabled to focus his attention: in other words, to channel his own attention into development or healing. An intriguing light has been cast on the quality of attention in healing by Magarey (1983) who argues that effective healers, whatever techniques they may use, have the ability to still their minds, to be calm, to extinguish their sense of separateness from others and to transmit this meditative state to their patients. We have argued in this book that, when the therapeutic relationship works well, the empathy between the practitioner and patient transforms the state of the patient, enabling him to mobilize his own healing energy.

WHAT DO PATIENTS EXPERIENCE AS HEALING?

Kleinman & Sung (1979) commented that healing is an embarrassing word for many clinicians, since it exposes the fundamental roots of medicine which have been buried under the technological advances of modern health care. They suggested that there are two separate healing functions: control of the disease and provision of meaning for the individual's experience of it. It seems that much modern technological medicine may achieve the first function, focused on cure, but that this leaves patients longing for the satisfaction of the second function through receiving care, comfort and understanding. Successful treatment in the eyes of the patient, as we have argued in Chapter 4, may require attention to the quality of care as well as to the clinical outcome.

Delin (1996) noted that there has been no systematic detailed enquiry into the essential elements of 'help' as experienced by those who seek help from alternative practitioners. She conducted a semi-structured interview with a small number of people who had sought help from medical or psychological practitioners at various stages in their lives, covering their experiences, perceptions, desires and ascribed meanings. 'Help' meant something different for each participant, including: provision of a regime of management, compassion, empowerment, information, explanation, caring, technical skills, honesty, respect and tolerance. Her conclusion concurs with the position put forward through this book:

Evidently, help-seekers strongly desire congruence between their construction of their problem and their needs and that of the helper, and a recognition of their uniqueness and their humanity. For some of the participants, it was almost as if their pursuit of help with their presenting physical or psychological problems was secondary, and that a desire for compassion and understanding in relation to their existential plight underlay their help-seeking. (Delin 1996: 9)

We must bear in mind the possibility that help in coming to grips with the meaning of life, or dealing with one's existential plight, may be secondary for those patients whose first priority is to deal quickly with acute or life-threatening suffering. Nevertheless, this desire or search for some sort of recognition of suffering and its meaning for the individual within his social context remains a constant theme throughout the literature on patients' perspectives on treatment.

Kleinman & Sung (1979) investigated the healing rituals used by shamanic folk healers in Taiwan. The authors described the healing ritual as having three definable stages. First, the patient's problem is named. Second, the appropriate ritual is performed to treat the problem, and herbs and practical advice are often given. The patient may be told that he is passing through a crisis. There may be ritualistic and ceremonial involvement of family and the patient's wider network. Third, the patient is told that he is healed. It is noted that this three-part division is typical of traditional healing rituals in many cultures and it parallels the process of much modern clinical care and psychotherapy.

The majority of those patients treated by shamanic healers, who were followed up by Kleinman & Sung, judged themselves to have been successfully treated, often using criteria which may be different from those of Western clinicians, including alleviation of distress in key family members, behavioural change, social benefits and psychological relief. Kleinman & Sung argued that indigenous practitioners are experienced by their patients as healing (even when, as in many cases, no objectively measurable change occurred in their symptoms) precisely because they are embedded in and involved with the social values and cultural expectations of their patients and thus the practitioners work to achieve the sorts of outcomes required and valued by their patients. In this book we have also argued that patients are often satisfied with complementary health care because, independently of its success in directly challenging their symptoms, it often meets patients' broader needs for explanation, empowerment and personal care. This has important implications for the evaluation of complementary health care.

RESEARCH INTO COMPLEMENTARY HEALTH CARE EFFECTIVENESS

Research about complementary therapy needs to take into account the holistic nature of treatment and to try to find out how the treatment process as a whole can be used to achieve the broad range of outcomes which patients want. A holistic approach to research requires a broad view of the entire research endeavour. Essentially, the term 'research' means 'to find out about' or 'to look again': systematic investigation towards increasing the sum of knowledge. Looking again means taking a fresh look at that which at first sight seems obvious: to question. The aim of research is to look at patients (their needs and wants, their health and their diseases, illnesses and sickness), ourselves, our knowledge and techniques with as little prejudice and preconception as possible. A holistic approach to research should lead to: broader and deeper attempts at understanding and explanation; empowerment of patients in the joint enterprise of treatment and evaluation; greater awareness of the impact of the therapeutic relationship; and increased knowledge of the technical and non-technical aspects of treatment in symptom reduction.

The traditional approach to scholarship has required impartiality, objectivity and disinterestedness while, on the other hand, we have seen that effectiveness in treatment is in part based on commitment, enthusiasm and belief. How can the practitioner, whose effective clinical practice appears to require a commitment to certain beliefs, put these on one side in order to pursue disinterested enquiry? Is it that the qualities needed for good researchers are incompatible with those needed for good clinicians? There are two answers to these questions. First, it is recognized now that no approach to knowledge and understanding can be neutral and value free: the challenge lies in acknowledging, rather than disregarding, biases and assumptions and questioning their implications for action and enquiry. Second, the overriding commitment, which unites the concerns of the researcher and the clinician, must be to honesty and integrity of approach. Both research and practice involve careful observation, some sort of formulation which relates observation, ideas and action, and honest appraisal of results.

The issue of scrutiny of results leads on to the next problem about research in practice. There is an increasing call for practitioners of all persuasions to demonstrate the effectiveness of treatment: in the NHS this is described as a demand for evidence-based medicine (Sackett et al 1996). In a world of limited resources, justice requires that public money should be spent on that health care which can be demonstrated to improve most efficiently the health status of the whole community (Culyer 1997). It is rightly the case that policy makers need to consider just and equitable bases for the distribution of resources.

The clinical trial, in which the impact of new treatment is compared with the impact of the best currently available treatment (or against 'placebo' treatment if no alternative is available) on similar groups of patients, is one method used to provide evidence of effectiveness. The randomized, double-blind clinical trial, in which patients are randomly assigned to the treatments being compared and in which neither patients nor clinicians know which treatment is being delivered, has been considered to be the most powerful test of effectiveness. This method is thought to rule out all possibility of systematic bias due to expectation of success or to pre-existing differences between patients receiving the different treatments. The relevance of clinical trials to complementary health care has been much debated; the problem is how to retain methodological rigour while also remaining true to the basic philosophical principles of health and healing (Mercer et al 1995).

Individual patients and individual practitioners are less immediately concerned with justice and impartiality than with individual need and partiality. People tend to want the best for themselves and for those they care about. Patients hope that practitioners, at least during their consultation, will be partial and do all within their power to meet their particular needs. Therefore, a practitioner is more likely to be concerned with the effectiveness of treatment for the individual patient with whom she is faced, rather than with efficient use of treatments for groups of patients or for the population overall. Large-scale clinical trials which look at the outcome of treatments for groups of patients are unlikely to be of immediate relevance for practitioners because the results of such trials tend to mask individual differences and may be generalized only to the highly specified conditions of the trial rather than the particular circumstances of the practitioner's treatment setting and the real-life situation of the patient. Individual practitioners want to know what treatment may be best suited to this particular person, with this particular set of difficulties, living in these particular circumstances and with these particular desired outcomes.

Large-scale trials have tended so far, to depend on generalized outcome measures which have usually been based on society's and professionals' collective views of the aims of treatment, which may not reflect the wants and needs of the individual patient. A further complication arises here too, because the wants, needs and desired outcomes are likely to change during the process of treatment in individual health care. Practitioners who wish to study the impact of their particular treatments need relevant, patient-centred outcome measures, which so far are in short supply.

Patients largely come to practitioners not because they know and understand evidence of effectiveness across groups but because they have had individual recommendations based on stories of effectiveness of treatments for individuals – often dismissed as 'anecdotal' evidence. We need to find ways of rigorously describing and checking the clinical significance of such stories. Here lies an opportunity for patients and practitioners to demonstrate that complementary health care may produce the sorts of outcomes which patients themselves most value. This is one of the means by which the incorporation of complementary approaches into the NHS may add to what Patrick Pietroni (1992) has called the 'greening of modern medicine', that is, acceptance of limits, sharing of power, demystification of the expert and increased awareness of patients' views.

THE PROCESS OF TREATMENT

We have argued most strongly in this book, particularly in Chapter 6, that healing is a social process, that the nature of change in expert healing is a special case of the way in which development is fostered within ordinary human relationships. Careful consideration of the nature of the so-called 'placebo effect' and 'spontaneous remission' requires us to reverse the more conventional understanding of the nature of expert help and to argue instead that the non-specific aspects of treatment are actually specifiable and, moreover, are central to healing.

The healing practitioner provides a setting in which the patient can collaborate with the practitioner about the aims and desired outcomes of treatment. The patient must feel safe within the treatment setting and with the practitioner. The patient can begin to feel more at ease when he senses that he is respected and genuinely cared for by the practitioner. Safety and security provide a framework within which the nature and meaning of the illness and of the treatment may be negotiated. The systematic use of ritual and ceremony facilitates concentration, strengthening the hope and belief that a positive outcome may be achieved. Therapeutic techniques, along with any healing ritual used, symbolize the power and magic of the healing process and can emphasize the special nature of the healing relationship. The therapeutic techniques may further offer comfort and relief and may in addition directly challenge the patient's symptoms and beliefs. The patient may be further empowered to manage his illness more effectively through following practical advice and by encouragement to use the personal and social resources available to him outside the treatment setting. Thus the patient is helped, when necessary, to change his feelings, thoughts, beliefs and behaviour in ways which raise his morale and which encourage him to cope actively with his situation. The person is treated as a whole person, whose life and experience are significant, meaningful and worthy of attention, who can be dependent for a while on the practitioner, yet who is also enabled to become autonomous.

The practitioner, too, through her active involvement and participation in healing, may use each encounter with a patient as an opportunity to facilitate her own continued development as a person. The ideal within treatment is to challenge the threatened chaos of illness and suffering and to transform it, through the joint process of integration and differentiation, into a manageable and meaningful experience. Thus, the therapeutic relationship provides a means of facilitating those growth-enhancing interactions which empower others and ourselves, to which we alluded in the first chapter.

The message of this book is that the nature of the healing task cannot be separated from the people undertaking that task. We hope that careful attention to the therapeutic relationship will give patients and practitioners alike the safety, care and challenge which will enable them to flourish in their own particular ways, as remarkable yet at the same time real and ordinary people. We hope, moreover, that practitioners will continue to strive to achieve the aims of the ancient aphorism on healing: to cure sometimes, relieve often and comfort always.

REFERENCES

Cassell E J 1978 The healer's art. Penguin, Harmondsworth
Csikszentmihalyi M 1992 Flow: the psychology of happiness. Rider, London
Culyer A J 1997 Maximising the health of the whole community. British Medical Journal 314:667–669
Delin C R 1996 An exploration of help-seekers' perceptions of the meaning of 'help'. Clinical Psychology Forum 94:26–29
Kleinman A, Sung L H 1979 Why do indigenous practitioners successfully heal? Social Science and Medicine 138:7–26
Magarey C 1983 Holistic cancer therapy. Journal of Psychosomatic Research 27:181–184
Mercer G, Long A F, Smith I J 1995 Researching and evaluating complementary therapies: the state of the debate. Nuffield Institute for Health, Leeds
Needleman J 1985 The way of the physician. Penguin, Harmondsworth
Pietroni P C 1992 Alternative medicine: methinks the doctor protests too much and incidentally befuddles the debate. Journal of Medical Ethics 18(1):23–25
Sackett D L, Richardson W S, Rosenberg W, Haynes R B (eds) 1996 Evidence-based medicine: how to practise and teach EBM. Churchill Livingstone, Edinburgh

Author Index

Subject Index